SECRET TO HUNZA SUPERIOR HEALTH

HOW PEOPLE OF HUNZA STAY YOUNG WITH EXTRAORDINARY HEALTH AND LIVE LONGER

By Carl Classic

Contributing Editor: Gordon F. Richiusa

Published by
Center for Human Natural Nutrition

Although the writer and publisher have extensively researched the source of any information provided herein to confirm its accuracy, authentication and completeness, we assume no responsibility for any inaccuracies, errors and omissions in the text of this book. Any slights of people or organizations are unintentional. Readers should use their own common sense and judgment and consult holistic or conventional medical experts to determine health care which is appropriate to each individual situation. We can accept no responsibility for any specific application to individual cases.

ISBN #0-9628298-7-0

Published by:

Center for Human Natural Nutrition
15015 Ventura Boulevard
Sherman Oaks, California 91403

First Printing 1989
Second Printing 1990
Third Printing 1991

Printed in the United States of America

Contents

Acknowledgement

I am deeply indebted to a great number of people who have aided me in many ways in the preparation of this book. I would especially like to thank those who were generous enough to share their personal experiences with natural, live foods for the Testimonials section. I am sorry that I was unable to use all the letters that were sent to me, and would like to make clear that those letters which you will be reading represent only a small selection of those that were received.

I am also deeply grateful to the individuals, including some close friends, who have tried the Hunza diet, and not only have experienced amazing results, but are now also dedicated advocates to the Hunza lifestyle.

IMPORTANT NOTICES

1. This manual is not intended to serve as a prescription for any ailment or as a substitute for professional medical care. Since we are not medical practitioners, we can not diagnose any disease or prescribe medication or treatment. The statements contained in this book express the opinions of the writer, based upon personal research.

2. But, it is our sincere belief that every human being who is in sound mental condition has the right to live the best possible life he can and to choose whatever method he thinks is best to heal his ailments. It is our right to choose between the conventional medicine (which is nothing but to inject our bodies with a host of chemicals, *reacting* to our health needs rather than trying to guide them) and the natural method, which is to improve your immune system (a God-given doctor within you) with High Quality Nutrition. In the end is not only our right, but our *duty* to let our immune system take care of us.

We believe that such right have been vested in us not only by the Constitution, but more importantly by our Creator.

We also understand that the medical profession takes such statements as direct challenges to their authority and don't like them. We, on the other hand, consider our statements (which you hear more often these days) as a direct challenge to a lucrative business, to take humanity into account before making prescriptions.

3. If, anywhere in the following text exercise is recommended or suggested, you should be aware that these are general recommendations, made for those who have been on live foods for more than a year and diagnosed to be in good health by health practitioners. If you are currently eating largely conventional foods, or have just changed your diet to natural, live foods, or have done no exercise for a long period of time, then we suggest that you first get a physical check-up to determine your fitness and establish a sensible timetable for your exercise program.

INTRODUCTION

Two of the oldest dreams of humanity have been the attainment of eternal life and happiness. In the literature of every modern civilization, and the oral traditions of most other cultures, the quest for happiness and long life have taken on mythic proportions. The Greeks and Romans had their Mt. Olympus and lucky was the occasional mortal who was granted access to the life-span of the gods. The Vikings looked forward to Valhalla, and the American Indians believed in the eternal Happy Hunting Grounds.

Even as our own culture was being forged, history records the actions of individuals who devoted their lives to the pursuit of elusive and (by today's standards) foolhardy goals such as the search for the Fountain Of Youth.

Often, these individuals who seek to prove the existence of the legendary, wreak the lives of all who come into contact with them. Sometimes these visionaries have been ruthless in their pursuits or sadly idealistic. In either case, they cannot achieve their goals and end up destroying others without a care, or are themselves destroyed as they try to attain the unattainable.

There are a few, however who have been motivated by more humane forces, wanting only to alleviate the ills and woes of the world. In this group, there is the even more rare individual who possesses this humanitarian quality as well as a clarity of mind; the dreamer who knows where the practical world ends and illusion begins.

Luckily, the ability to dream and seek is a quality that has remained with the human spirit. Today, many great minds are still driven by a desire to fulfill these lofty human needs. All go about their quests in varying ways, using every imaginable method. But, the truth is, each of us, in some way is affected by the pursuit of happiness and long life. The two goals, in fact are closely interrelated and a part of human nature.

If you, for instance, are a hard working person who tries to stay healthy merely so that you might live a little longer, so that you will have a better chance of attaining personal wealth for your family, then your final aim is really happiness. But that happiness is directly linked to extending your life. You may even have 'calculated' your life to be a certain number of years as a requirement to achieve your goals. The interesting thing is that HEALTH is merely a by-product of the plan toward happiness.

There is nothing wrong with seeking personal happiness, or with making it a prime objective in life. Remember, the 'pursuit of happiness' is one of the inalienable rights that the authors of the U.S. Constitution saw fit to include in a place of prominence in the Preamble of our own Bill Of Rights.

But, with all the importance that people seem to place on it, we must wonder how humanity arrived at this goal as something with so much importance, even more important than Health. Is it that mankind has been caught in an intellectual dilemma, trying to decide if these two goals should be prime objectives?

No, this is simply not so. These two dreams (long life and happiness) have come to the minds of men instinctively, without any interference from our intellect. This instinct has been built into every living cell, separate from our conscious thought processes.

But, the major mistake is that our 'instinctive desires' are rooted in an even 'Higher Power'. We are driven, we believe, by a **responsibility** that was bestowed upon us at creation. This responsibility was expressed in the Old Testament when God charged Adam with dominion over his environment. This was a classic 'Two Edged Sword', in that we both could dominate the earth, by virtue of our intelligence and inherent nature, but must also CARE FOR NATURE and all other creatures upon the earth. Forgetting this directive from our Creator is the single most reason we have been unable, as a race, to achieve the goals which we've just mentioned.

Scientists and Sages alike have spent countless hours and endless energy looking for single answers to these Ultimate Questions. Countless journeys have been made, millions of miles traveled in search of the elixirs that provide long life and happiness.

Therein lies the problem. For, whenever we take even a single step in our search and look outward, we are looking in the wrong place. The answer is and has always been within. This may sound corny or 'too simple' to many who might read these lines, but to prove what we are saying we need merely to look at the smallest parts of ourselves, our individual cells. Each of our own tiny cells is a complete, living entity with an intelligence and 'driving force' all its own. They possess, in other words, a 'will to survive'. They are separate units, free (in a sense) from our intellectual choices...and yet, each of these microscopic organisms is endowed with the same two goals that have become the Dreams of Mankind. They have also been granted a sense of **'responsibility'**. Each cell 'knows' instinctively that if the 'body' does not survive then the individual is lost as well. Everything is dependent upon everything else, then. From the other end of the proposition, if we take care of ourselves and follow the rules of creation, then the whole 'body' will prosper and our goals for **long life and happiness will be attainable.**

Think of it this way: each cell is constantly in the process of reproducing itself 'according to its own kind'. New, healthy cells are created so that life can be extended for as long as possible. In addition, these single cells combine together in a number of miraculous ways to form the various chemicals, systems and organs of the body. These organs and other separate units do their individual instinctive best to survive and to make life as pleasant as possible for the body as a whole.

If the weather is hot, for example, certain cells, and systems make the determination to produce perspiration in an attempt to cool the entire organism. The body (as a whole) even goes so far as to cool some parts more or less than others, depending upon their own preferences, needs and abilities. And, remember, this all happens AUTOMATICALLY, without your ever having to think about it. Each individual cell and organ seems to know its **responsibility** and that by **working together each and all will benefit.**

As incredible as this interaction is, our main point is simple. This kind of reaction, this striving for a happier and longer life is rooted in all our instincts even to our very smallest and subconscious parts.

There is one very important conclusion that we can reach from all that we have said. The conclusion is that our CREATOR'S and NATURE'S intention for life on this planet has always been the pursuit of a longer and happier life. This principle, from the very beginning of creation, has been rooted and programed into the fabric of every living cell imbued with life by our creator.

A natural kind of question then is, **can we truly improve our chances of staying alive longer and being happier?**

Answering this question is really what this book is all about. **It is possible to live longer and happier lives,** we believe. But, first we must make the effort to rearrange our thinking somewhat. We cannot, like the seekers of the past, achieve these goals at the cost of other lives...since we know that ALL must benefit for each of us to truly prosper.

In our pursuit of happiness and longer life we cannot think of health as an 'extra added attraction'. The truth is that happiness and long life are mere by-products of healthy nutrition, lifestyle and other physical habits. It is not the other way around.

Most importantly, we believe that this book will appeal to you on more than one level, because the answers you will read here will not only make sense to your intellect, but will satisfy the instinctual desires that dwell in every cell of your body.

An interesting oriental proverb states something very similar to what Jesus said to his disciples about the voice of the Holy Spirit. The saying goes,"The truth is already in all humans, ready to answer all questions. One needs only to ask IS THIS THE TRUTH? And, the inner voice will answer, every time, quickly, precisely giving you proper guidance. The problem is that very few ask."

By buying this book, we believe that you will have the opportunity of asking your inner self an important question. By reading it and allowing yourself an opportunity to 'think for yourself,we further believe and hope that **you will finally find your own Fountain of Youth, your Elixir of Happiness.**

CHAPTER ONE

WORDS OF GOD...

And the Lord God formed man from the dust of the ground and breathed into his nostrils for breath of life."
        --Genesis 2:7
"...And the Lord God planted a garden in Eden, away to the east, and there he put the Man whom he had formed. The Lord God made trees spring from the ground, all trees pleasant to look at and good for food...God also said, 'I give you all plants that bear seed everywhere on earth and every tree bearing fruit which yields seed: They shall be yours for food.'"
        --Genesis 2:8 and 1:29

These quotes from scripture represent the most fundamental principles of human life on earth which have been ignored and overlooked for so long that they are now completely forgotten. No one in this age refers to these verses as guidelines for human nourishment and lifestyle, whereas the wisdom in these verses is a clear directive to man for his food and living environment.

It is clearly indicated that we are created from nature and should live and be nourished by nature.

According to scripture, "God formed man from the dust of the ground". What this simply means is that human beings are created from nature and are an integral part of the earth. They come from earth and they will, one day be returned to the earth.

Genesis 2:8 and 1:29, say "God planted a garden (nature)......... and there He put the Man whom He had formed." In the same quote God specifies what shall be man's food. Nowhere in this quote do we see any mention of conventional foods, either the kind being eaten at the time when the scripture was written or the present conventional food.

God could have made anything for man to live on or to eat. Being all powerful has that kind of advantages, but there must have been a wisdom of placing him in nature (the Garden) and directing him to use nature (plants that bear seed anywhere on earth and every tree bearing fruit which yields seed) for his nourishment. But, knowledge in this case also required wisdom, something that Humans are not well known for. God knew that humans would need to be reminded of their responsibilities to the earth. For that reason, HE (God) planted a garden, a place that would require that humans STAY DIRECTLY INVOLVED with Nature and the process of life.

What's more natural than a garden? And, what kind of food supply would keep humans directly involved with the processes, and forces of life? A garden with LIVING FOOD, by far, was the best idea for a place to live, and for growing food to eat.

What this all boils down to is that human being come from nature and can only live and thrive within the confines of nature.

The creation of the natural laws which include the workings of the whole earth with its minerals, plants, animals, and human beings is a work of perfection and an endless fascination for us.

Today's science might argue with some minute point in religion, but everyone agrees whole heartedly with the conclusion we have just made.

Today, 2000 years (or more) since the time that the scriptures were being written, the latest scientific research proves the accuracy of these words of wisdom. In a later chapter of this book, under the sub-heading AIR, you will read the latest scientific research by NASA's environmental research lab at the John C. Stennis Space Center in Mississippi. This research proves that plants are the best means of cleaning, purifying, refreshing and revitalizing your indoor air. The research suggests placing indoor plants, as many as possible, into your home environment, possibly changing your indoors into a garden, itself.

On the nutrition side of things, research in recent years, has concluded that for a healthier, longer and more active life we should eat more.fruits, vegetables, grains and seeds. Even the American Heart Association, American Cancer Society and the Academy of Sciences who until a few years ago were denying any link between diet and heart disease or cancer, now have gone half-way, recommending (only) to increase our intake of foods rich in fiber and low in fat such as fruits, vegetables, grains and cereals.

Even with todays changes in scientific opinion we honestly believe that because of very close connection of the business world (the industry -specially the health industry) and the world of science, the scientist (who is serving both worlds - and most scientists are in that position) can not and will not tell us the whole truth.

It is ironic and somewhat foolish when we hear about thousands of "scientists" working around the clock "claiming" that they are "improving" the work of perfection, the natural order of things.

We could name thousands of examples where so called "scientists" claim, they have either improved the performance of nature or they are researching ways of making 'life a little better'. How can we improve perfection, though? Here are a few ways that "Science" has tried...and failed.

Many years ago, there was a major effort made by the Scientific Community to improve Mother's Milk by creating a 'balanced' formula milk powder. This push was so strong and the advertising so convincing that for decades almost every mother who could afford it, fed their infants prepared formula. Today, the true scientist will tell you that there is nothing close to natural mother's milk for an infant. Any animal milk or the best baby formula ever made by man will never compare to what the Creator gave to us for free.

The sad fact is that science is now telling us that some diseases in childhood and most of our illnesses and short comings in later life can be directly related to the baby formulas. Is this how they have improved the work of mother nature? Have these same scientists forgotten that it was they who gave us the 'false nutrition' in the first place?

Another example of mistaken human pride, can be seen in the past claim that with chemicals (fertilizers) we might produce bigger apples or oranges or other kinds of fruits and vegetables. For years we dumped every conceivable chemical and unnatural substance into the soils and on the growing plants. The fruits and vegetables did get bigger. What they didn't tell us however is that the nutritional value of these foods that we once counted on as completely nutritious, had dropped in value to only a fraction of what an unpolluted, organically grown apple, orange or vegetable would be. In other words, the apple you get as a result of commercial growing is not the apple which spawned the old saying, "an apple a day keeps the doctor away".

In fact , a recent 'about-face' by these same scientists has concluded that there are now so many chemicals in our apples (in the form of pesticides and absorbed chemicals from fertilizers) that we can expect the doctor will become a very close friend, since you will have to visit him regularly if you intend to EAT these large, apples which contain very little nutrition.

Is this improving the work of mother nature? If you still are unable to answer this question, let's look at one final example of the blundering of modern man. Today's big news stories all seem to center around medical "scientists", working around the clock to improve our health and vitality. Our immune mechanism, this natural system of the wonderful machine (the human body) has been placed within us to work as a natural defense system, as well as a natural healing mechanism. Scientists on the other hand want to rid you of diseases (after you've got them) by injecting chemicals into your body, or prevent them in the same, unnatural way. This concept has also been proven a total failure.

We know this for a fact, because with all the bragging about "advancements" in "medical science" and doing "miracles" we have not stopped the increase in the prevalence of disease. The quantity and variety of diseases, during the past 50 years has been increasing by the day (not the other way around as some would have you believe). And, what is worse is that due to millions of tons of different prescription and over the counter drugs (chemicals) shoved into the general public's systems, the quality of life, physically and mentally has deteriorated to an all time low.

The individuals who claim to be "scientists" and try to interfere with the ecology and the orderly processes of nature in the name of improving the work of the Creator are nothing but a bunch of cheap businessmen trying to achieve personal wealth at the cost of human health.

Finally, our message to these so called "scientists" is, "Please, stop interfering in nature, a work of perfection." The human body and Mother Earth still have the ability to repair themselves. These safety measures were also built into the system.

The Creator needs no one to improve His work. Human effort that is focused on improving the Natural Processes is not going to help humanity. Instead these desires will create more unfavorable conditions, which will result in pain and suffering. Mr. or Ms. Scientist, we feel that the human body, the earth and for that matter all of NATURE are gifts given to us by the Creator. They belong to all of us, and it is our right to ask you to stop interfering in their orderly processes.

CHAPTER TWO

A RETURN TO NATURAL LOGIC

Congratulations! By purchasing this book and beginning to read it, you've shown yourself to be a special breed of person. Your initiative has proven your willingness to take responsibility for improving the conditions of your life. You are a very select and special person.

You've also shown yourself to possess an open mind, and the invaluable trait of being able to consider a concept fully and completely, before you make a judgment about it (or reject it because it is different from your conventional way of thinking). Another important characteristic that we assume you possess is that you place your mental and physical health high up on your list of priorities. This trait, we are thankful, appears to be on the increase in our country. More and more persons are looking for ways (such as you are) to get fit or 'into better shape' and we applaud everyone who has helped in the effort to reshape our 'collective health consciousness'.

We have established ourselves as a focal point for this new energy. We wanted to create a Center of information for the Health Conscious, as well as a link between those who have information and those who desperately want and need it.

This book is a major culmination of our efforts. We have taken a great deal of time, and put a lot of effort into the production (including research, testing and preparation) of **SECRET TO HUNZA SUPERIOR HEALTH**.

Our aim, now, is the same as it was when we started the ball rolling. We want to reach the kind of person that you are with a true and honest message about endless energy, freedom from disease and long, happy life that may seem revolutionary to some, even though much of what we first published many years ago (as medical blasphemy) is now commonplace and widely accepted.

We are proud to say that we did not wait for the medical world to 'catch up' to what our **'inner voice'** told us was the truth. We are sure, from countless letters delivered from our readers, that we've helped a good number of people. Some of those persons would probably not be here today, if they had not learned a new and workable way to excellent health and a longer, happier life.

So, while the concepts in this book might still seem revolutionary to some, that is only because one is looking at these concepts from an unhealthy perspective. Remember, good health is only a radical idea from the point of view of 'popular opinion'.

The concepts in this book are based on long historical precedent. And, we will prove, by unraveling a number of persistent, twisted and distorted facts (and by presenting the latest statistics and documentation) that the goal of **SUPREME HEALTH CAN BE YOURS**.

In addition to all the statistics and logical conclusions that we draw from our own investigations, we will supply you with a number of true life narratives, testimonials of individuals in our own society as well as a factual account of an entire community of people to show you how these highly prized ambitions can be a reality in your very own life. You've just taken the first step on an important journey. And, the first step is always the most important.

THE HISTORY OF FREE THINKING

Although modern human history is relatively brief, by comparison, we have, as a race, been remarkably consistent in one respect. Whenever someone presented a new idea, or was willing to listen to their 'inner voice' or the logic of a new concept they were usually met with scorn, ridicule and sometimes punishment.

In today's world, even the youngest child accepts the logic, for instance, of the earth and other planets orbiting around the sun. Yet, when men like Copernicus and Galileo first introduced this idea and the concepts that are interrelated to it, they were met with exactly the kinds of responses from the general public and the educated, scientific communities that we've just listed.

The sad irony is that their ideas were the first logical responses to long, unanswered questions about the workings of the Universe and our position in the cosmos. Until the time of Copernicus, people (that's EDUCATED people) truly believed things like the world was flat and that it was held in place by four large elephants on the back of a gigantic turtle. It was years, however, before the ideas of men like Copernicus and Galileo caught on, and decades before the Educated community accepted for fact what an eight year old child never questions today.

But, this is the way humanity has always worked, first to be frightened of the new and unusual, to base their beliefs on their fears and ignorance, to oppose the truth when it is presented and finally, (when the truth is made obvious through honest evaluation) to embrace the new idea and pretend that it was always known.

In the area of human health it has not been any different. Not too many years ago it was a 'well known fact' that a healthy diet consisted of a good portion of meat and very little carbohydrates. Today, of course, we know that this is all wrong. Every day new evidence is uncovered to support the 'new truth' that meat (especially red meat) is literally counter-healthy.

So, the facts we grew up with do not always turn out to be the 'truth'. We never thought to question the teachings of our parents and they never thought to question the teachings of their mothers and fathers. The problem is that what our parents were teaching us about health and happiness was not based on what they 'knew to be true', but on what they had been told to accept as truth. Many people undoubtedly felt the need for changes in our human health standard, but to oppose the routines of society meant ridicule and perhaps even death. Forcing change on an unwilling social order was not really worth the trouble.

How did we allow our health standards to come to be based on false beliefs, rather than what we knew, in our hearts, to be true? More importantly, is it possible to change things from the way that they once were? Please read on.

A RETURN TO COMMON SENSE

The true worth of an idea lies, not it the dollar value we place upon it, but in its benefit to mankind and the Earth on which we live. These benefits are measured in the amount of health and happiness they bestow. Doing the RIGHT thing does not necessarily mean financial benefit (in fact, the two are usually exclusive of one another).

Now, we must ask ourselves what is the best way of making a judgment on the benefits of an idea or a theory? There are three ways of examining the accuracy of any new or even an old idea.

The first (and by far the most tried and true method) is by experience.   Although, this is the best way of determining somethings' value, it could require a very lengthy period of time. Time, especially when dealing with your health, is not something that you have a lot of. The fact is, you might run out of time before your experience shows you enough information. Also, some of the effects of your experiences will come to light many tens of years after the fact. Let me give you an example.

If you are a moderate smoker or drinker you might enjoy what you are doing at the time and feel very little or no effect on your health. But the real adverse side-effects will come to light many years later. And, this is not all.

There is another problem in trying to judge by experience. Let's assume that someone has a terminal disease and the doctor recommends surgery or chemotherapy or both. Let us assume that, because of fear of death, the patient decides to experience the doctor's recommendation. What if, at a later date the patient finds out he has made the wrong decision. How can he bring back the organ which was separated from his body and thrown away? How can you undo the sever adverse effects of chemotherapy?

The old saying then, "there is no teacher like experience" might be true, but short term experiences could be very misleading. A pain killer, for instance will give an immediate relief to your headache but not only will it not solve the real problem, it will also leave you to suffer more adverse effects in the long run.   The immediate relief might seem like a positive result (at the time), but there is very few substances that destroy the stomach lining the way that aspirin does.

There is another way of examining the value of a belief then. This is through the scientific method. This method (although the most highly respected) is the most misleading way of judging something for the simple reason that "Scientists" (the ones who are going to examine the belief and conduct the research) are not really interested in 'pure research' (as they would have us believe) but are engaged in serving a phase of our conglomerate industry. Almost all "Scientists" (for personal gains) are serving the Big Business Industry, and their interpretation of the research will usually have a tendency of favoring the hand that feeds them."

What we are simply saying is that almost every so called "Scientist" is in some way associated with a industrial or financial institute and his prime responsibility is to protect the interest of that institute in order to maintain his job.

This statement excludes some real scientists who's research is based solely on humanitarian goals. Certainly, they need financing, but the financial interests will not effect their findings. Imagine a scientist working for a nuclear energy company telling the public that nuclear energy is definitely harmful or a dangerous proposition.

There are even "Scientists" (researchers) working for the Tobacco industry trying to introduce new methods of safe smoking or "Scientists" working for meat industry trying to prove the importance of animal protein for human health.

So, this method of inquiry has its problems. But, there is another way for us to test an idea's worth.

Again, we must heed our inner voice. But, what exactly is the inner voice and how do we get to it? The answer is simple. The inner voice has always been available to us, in fact, it is known by another name...**our common sense.**   This sense we have is our best way of telling if something is truly good and valuable to us. It's our most powerful tool for survival, yet, because of modernization it is a tool that has long been unused.

That is where we get the joke, "if common sense is so common, then why doesn't anyone have it?" The reality is that we ALL 'have', but we seldom **USE** it.

We all have the power within us to decide if something is good and true. Generally, our 'gut' feelings are proven to be correct. But, humans are social creatures who are driven more by the group pressures that surround them, than they are by the voice from within. If only we would listen to our 'voice' and ignore what others are telling us, we'd be much better off.

Remember, what we are saying is not blasphemy. Every great sage, including Jesus told us how simple it was to achieve miracles. All we have to do is speak and listen to 'the spirit whose voice comes from within.' The answers are always true and will always be available.

With this book, we will try and reverse a resent, modern trend of ignoring the Voice From Within and 'relearn' how to use our Common Sense. The result, we believe is that endless, new horizons will unfold for you.

Our method is simple and straight forward. We will try to encourage you to listen to your Common Sense (the voice within) and then, for assurance, double check it with the experience of others where you won't endanger your own health in gaining the experience. And, when we quote experiences we refer to the experiences of individuals in our own community, as well as communities with many hundreds of years of history to draw conclusions from. In the case of Hunza, this general body of experiences encompasses 2000

THE JOURNEY TOWARD SUCCESS

In the next few chapters we will attempt to present a number of ideas that will help enlighten you and guide you on a path toward incredible health, endless energy, freedom from disease and a long and happy life. We will make our suggestions in adherence to the laws of Nature that have been assigned to us by the Creator. Some ideas will seem new and revolutionary, some will appear commonplace. It is not so much how new a single idea is that is important, but the fact that each new idea (or old) is taken in consideration of the whole picture. And, we will NEVER say anything just to give you an answer to a mathematical problem. Our answers come from the heart and are made to benefit humanity. With this purpose in mind, armed with our Common Sense, and backed up with the experiences of others we cannot fail to supply you with a invaluable OVERALL APPROACH unlike anything you've ever seen before.

If the methods we suggest and the ideas expressed here meet with your criteria for Common Sense and logic, then your course of action should be clearly marked for you.

As a first test, we'd like you to ask yourself one simple question: "What is the one most important thing in a person's life?"

We believe that the answer most often received (if our Common Sense is activated) relates to our health. It doesn't matter if a person is rich or poor, highly placed or the poorest pauper on the streets. If you don't have your physical and mental health, then you really don't have anything, at all of value.

Isn't it funny how many REALLY RICH people end up dying because of their obsession with health? Look at Howard Hughes, for instance. He was cut off from enjoying the value of his vast wealth simply because he became obsessed with his health. His fatal flaw was that, instead of looking to common sense for his answers he relied on his money to save him. Science or Wealth are not the answers, they are merely other tools that we can possess. But, they are not THE one tool that we've all been granted by the Creator. And that is the one we **MUST** use. For, if a person does NOT use his Common Sense in determining a health plan for his life, then he will never achieve health. And, without health he can never enjoy his other discoveries (or his wealth) to the fullest.

A common belief is that the mind and body are separate, but we feel that it is totally obvious that physical and mental health are completely interrelated. To talk about one as opposed to the other is foolish, and to think of obtaining one at the expense of the other can lead only to ruin.

We'd like to point out, when we say TOTAL HEALTH we mean "the best possible health that an individual can obtain." We understand that genetics and even physical injury can play a roll in what one can achieve. If you are in a wheelchair due to handicaps of one kind or another, we know that you might never walk again. However, you can achieve Optimum Health on a personal level. You can, in other words, 'be the best you can possibly be'. And, that is what we want every person to achieve.

We assume that you (by buying this book) agree with this basic principle and are willing (if not eager) to take the responsibility for your own health into your own hands. We hope, also, that you see that you will need to begin seeing yourself as part of a total 'health environment'...a picture of health that includes a healthy world (the body of which we are a part). It is a well known fact that coming to any journey or task with a positive attitude and clear idea of our long and short term goals can assure success from the start.

THE ULTIMATE TEST

When we make our claims for Ultimate Health, later in this book we do not do so lightly or on the basis of faulty or unfounded evidence. Our claims are made according to the premise and the TEST of Common Sense. We will draw our conclusions from true-life experiences of actual human beings who are surviving and prospering according to our principles and are achieving amazing results. Our 'laboratory' is not a small room filled with mice, rabbits and monkeys. Our scientists are not separated from humanity, serving special interests or some large corporations.Our scientists begin their search by seeing themselves as an integral part of the Natural Environment. They do not base their findings on a few short tests performed on helpless animals. Our answers are derived from the laboratory of primitive, as well as, Modern Life. Our test tubes are our own bodies. Our 'control group' is a living community of individuals who have all the health benefits that we've listed above, including **mental, physical and sexual vitality** up to and beyond the **age of 100!**

What we will be talking about is the food we eat, the water we drink,the air we breathe and the physical activities we engage in. We will try and keep our total environment in perspective, and will demonstrate how all the life sustaining elements are ultimately responsible also for our mental and emotional state of being. In this way, our physical body affects every aspect of our lives.

In short, our main objective is to help you to achieve that most important goal of all humanity...Optimum Health and a longer, happy life.

The Ultimate Test does not lie in any statistic or scientific authority. The final verdict on what we say will come from your ability to utilize what you learn and apply it to your own life. Our goal at the Center For Human Natural Nutrition is dependent on your personal goals, then. For, our success will be measured, in part, by the success you feel within your own body. We will succeed **ONLY** if you do. So, we sincerely want you to succeed.

For this reason we will be as thorough as possible, without being tedious and boring. We've learned a lot over the years of giving our message, so those of you who have read some of our publications before will gain the full benefit of what we've learned by getting the whole story in one volume.

Like that sage advice that Dorothy was given in THE WIZARD OF OZ, "It's always best to start at the beginning." So, that's where we will begin.

When we conclude our journey together, we are convinced that you will have all the necessary tools to succeed in any action that you choose to take according to the principles presented.

CHAPTER THREE

EVOLUTION OF HUMAN NUTRITION
(The Hands Of Man...)

Regardless of what you may think of the many scientific disciplines, most accepted evidence of man's prehistoric existence points to certain conclusions.   Before the Modern Age, the time when human beings began to actively alter their environment, they were a functional part of the natural world. They flowed with the forces of nature, evolved within and were governed by the natural laws laid down by our CREATOR.

Because they were still true Children of God, innocent and essentially pure, all their needs were provided for in the same way that ALL creatures were taken care of.

When people were close to nature, they were continually involved in the physical activity of living and staying alive. Their only task, in other words, was simple survival. The rules were simple too, and were followed by all as a matter of course. You either followed the rules of nature or died.

At this time in mankind's existence, our main concerns were gathering food, rearing young and protecting the group from other, dangerous creatures. It was a time of basic needs and basic solutions. There was no disease. There was no tooth decay or heart attacks, or Cancer. Humans slept when they were tired and arose at the first light of dawn, since there was no artificial light (there was no artificial ANYTHING for that matter). And, there was no use of fire. Our only experience with this basic elemental reaction was when we witnessed an occasional lightning burn or prairie blaze.

The sun was the only permanent source of light or energy that was used freely by humans and everything else. That beautiful object in the sky gave life to all living plants and animals on the planet, and came to us in the perfect, proper amounts...there was no fear of melanoma (fatal skin cancers).

The reason that the sun contacted us in perfect quantities is that ALL the elements were untouched and in harmony with one another. And, WE were in harmony with them.

Certainly, there were fluctuations, but when changes occurred, the natural processes were more than adequate to rebalance the life-giving qualities of the Earth. In times of drought, fewer animals were born, people migrated, trees grew slower. When more oxygen was needed, the earth burst anew with fresh greenery that already flourished everywhere upon the planet like a beautiful, living cloak.

Most importantly, at this time in our history, Mankind nourished himself solely according to the laws of nature. We ate and drank what was already available in abundance. "The Lord God planted a garden in Eden....." and God also said, " I give you all plants that bear seed everywhere on earth and every tree bearing fruit which yields seed. They shall be yours for food".

Thirst was quenched with clean, fresh, live water, and every source of it was safe. Wastes were all natural, in manageable amounts and had not destroyed this basic element.

Hunger and nutritional needs were satisfied with green leaves, growing vegetables, fruits, grains, seeds and nuts. Man ate a proper balance and variety, as he moved from place to place or the seasons changed and the cycle of life continued around him. The soils were clean and unpolluted, giving forth nutrients rather than poisons.

The air too, was clean and fresh, as there were no man-made substances to interfere with any aspect of life...human or otherwise. It also was abundant and, as the web of life was in tact, it properly affected other important parts of our atmosphere (such as the Ozone Layer).

The most important element of man's existence at this glorious time in pre-history was his supreme health, which he took for granted as a result of his harmonious, natural life-style.

Humans were truly admirable creations, possessing the highest levels of vitality, intelligence and ability. They never suffered from headaches, influenza, insomnia, blood pressure problems, cancers, heart disease, arthritis, anxiety or any other ailment that Modern People have grown accustomed to.

DISEASE AND 'NORMAL' HEALTH
(To Be Or Not To Be.....Healthy)

Today, we have been led to believe that disease and ailment is a normal part of everyday life. In modern life, ill-health is common and good health is considered almost a miracle. A common greeting is to ask, "Is everyone well?" This seems polite, but points out our expectation of disease. And, this expectation holds true for every person at every age and stage of development. We have even taken to categorizing certain diseases according to the TIME that we should expect to get them. Some diseases are 'childhood' ones. Others are more common among the old and infirm; while still more should be expected to hit us during that 'gray period of time when we are 'going through the change and are slowing down.' This kind of statement is an example of that 'twisted logic' that we discussed earlier. It is also the kind of logic that allows us to accept diseases such as A.I.D.S. as a perverted kind of payment for our lazy, unnatural way of life. In other words, to paraphrase the old saying "if you're gonna play, you gotta pay", or "if you're going to live outside the laws of nature, you're going to get sick and die prematurely."

We know, simply speaking, that this is NOT TRUE, we do not need to expect or accept disease. Our belief, in fact, is that human beings have the capacity to be healthy throughout their **entire lives**.

In a coming chapter we will give you details of a community of people who have the good luck to exist in a remote area of the world and enjoy a very natural lifestyle. We also will give you accounts of individuals in our own Modern Society who have made a conscious choice to live more naturally. For both sets of persons (the remote community and those among us who correct what they can in their own lives), freedom from disease is a benefit that they take for granted. They live and (most importantly) EAT healthy and, consequently EXPECT and receive health as a by-product of their actions.

We believe that if conditions were made right, it would be possible for **everyone to** be graced with the same miraculous health and longevity as those in this small community who **live strong and happy lives to** ages of upwards of **ONE HUNDRED YEARS**.

THE ICE AGE: HUMAN HEALTH'S TURNING POINT

It is speculated by some scientists that the first drastic deviation from the wisdom of nature came with the onset of the Ice Age. We must note here that, until this time, mankind had used his amazing ability to build and shape things in a very simple and non-destructive manner. There was no need to make many changes, because everything that humans needed was supplied freely by nature. Living according to the laws of nature, mankind was, in a sense, at the mercy of nature as well. We survived and died according to the natural processes that we were a part of. But, we HAD the ability to manipulate things. The reason that we didn't manipulate things was that we didn't NEED to. We didn't change our habits because we didn't NEED to change them.

Then came the Ice Age (one of many that preceded it, but humanity's first experience with it), a period of sudden, extreme climatic change. Other species became extinct or migrated swiftly, or flew south. Humans were relatively slow and lazy. We couldn't fly and extinction was out of the question, so we did what we did best. We used our hands and we adapted. Since live natural food was no longer available to us. We started eating animal flesh only for survival, then over a longer period of time because of conditioning, meat became a part of our staple diet.We also realized the need to stay warm, so it is no surprise that at this time; mankind became skilled in the making of fire.

These two new abilities (killing and making fire) were both impressive to us and we not only surrounded each with elaborate rituals but quickly related these activities to one another. As the smell of raw meat was not very pleasing to human senses, and the meat was difficult to chew, we mixed the meat with vegetables and spices to change the taste. Cooking also made it easier to chew. At a later time we also found out that by burning the meat we could preserve it longer. We were, undoubtedly very impressed with ourselves.

But, if you think about it, this just made the prospect of eating flesh that much worse. Not only were we surviving on meat (which was a sudden and therefore unnatural addition to our long established diets) but we were burning it first, thus destroying almost all of its nutritional value.

We will substantiate later that man's digestive tract **IN NO WAY** corresponds to that of any other known carnivore. But, here, let it suffice to say that suddenly, the natural 'live foods' that humans had been conditioned by nature to flourish on (over a period of eons) was changed to include very little else but devitalized animal flesh and other 'altered' substances that were never intended for him.

THE FOUR HISTORICAL STAGES OF HUMAN NUTRITION

At the risk of being too simple, we are going to summarize man's nutritional history by establishing four stages or 'checkpoints'. The first stage, **AGE OF**

NATURAL NUTRITION we have already outlined. This was the longest and most important period of man's development, which began with human's first appearance on earth (about 1,500 million years ago by most estimates) and continued to the advent of the ICE AGE. It is imperative to our discussion that we realize this is the era when humans developed into their present physical form. They developed their needs, physically, mentally and emotionally. We established ourselves as a species and self awareness was beginning to set us apart from the other creatures. It is difficult to comprehend that span of time...1,500 MILLION YEARS! To compare, our present period of recorded history is extremely brief, spanning only few thousand years.

The second important stage in our development we will call **THE AGE OF ANIMAL FLESH**. We have discussed how the ICE AGE was integral in setting the stage for this period. The important contribution of this segment of time in the history of mankind occurs as a result of the eating of animal flesh (in some cases ONLY meat). When we took this turn away from our natural nutritional path, the health, energy and vitality of an essentially very fit species (mankind) began to deteriorate. As yet, we had not totally destroyed our environment (we had good water, air and soil), and we still performed many vital functions toward staying healthy (we got much more natural exercise), but the Building Blocks for human disease were all in place.

The development of our taste for cooked food also led us directly to the third stage of human nutrition, we call **THE COOKING AGE**. Humans became more proficient in (and impressed with) their ability to use fire. The ICE AGE ended and the need to migrate for hunting purposes no longer existed. Mankind, probably responding to his natural instincts, began to 'settle down' and to colonize. For a time, to a limited degree, mankind tried to reestablish his link with nature by farming the lands on which he lived. But, due to many years of establishing the importance of fire he also began to bake, roast, toast, and grill the life (literally) out of ALL the food that he once took directly from the earth and consumed LIVE, WHOLE AND COMPLETE nutritionally. Cooking everything, meant the destruction of all the nutritional elements of a diet that the human physiology had developed on. In fact, these elements had MADE humans what they were, they were vital to our health.

Again, instinct told us that things were not right. We could tell by the taste, smell and texture of meat that it was not natural to consume. But, we did not heed our inner voice, our voice of Common Sense. Instead, we added spices to our animal flesh and other cooked foods in an attempt to make them taste more like the natural foods our bodies unconsciously knew we needed.

Due to our obsessive nature and an uncanny ability to be impressed with ourselves, we viewed food preparation in the same way we once looked at fire-making. A variety of recipes developed. People even went to war over the differing ways that they prepared food.

All this interest in cooking and food preparation had two very logical conclusions. First, food addictions resulted. And, secondly, by adding herbs and spices to our foods for unnatural reasons the door was opened for the next and most fatal age of all.

The fourth stage (the one we are currently in) of human nutritional development we call the **AGE OF CHEMICALS**. This is a natural outgrowth of the age that preceded it and it laid the groundwork for an era where business interests have become the last word in the development of society. Common Sense, when voiced, is all but ignored. And, because of our own vanity, it is in the last one hundred years or so that most of our present, tragic situations have come to pass.

For, the AGE OF CHEMICALS has taken us completely (as a race) away from the harmony with nature which is necessary for any (individual) beings to survive. Remember, the law of Nature is precise: The body MUST survive if the cells are going to do the same. By allowing business interests to guide our lives, we have ignored our inner voice and allowed the alteration of every element of our once natural and completely nurturing environment. We've polluted our air, our water and can almost not even find live, healthy food to eat. No longer do our bodies receive the nourishment that was once so carefully provided by nature. Therefore, few (if any) of our physiological needs are met. And, due to an unnatural life-style, separate from the natural laws, none of our psychological, mental or emotional needs (established in the millions of years of pre-history) are met either.

Instead, in the AGE OF CHEMICALS, with the prompting and cooperation of business, we succeeded in substituting almost ALL natural elements with unnatural, man-made, chemical replacements which in no REAL sense resemble the living elements that they are supposed to replace. Just because a plastic orange LOOKS like an orange, doesn't mean it's really an orange.

In the end, what this means is that man has changed his entire environment, but is basically the same creature, with the same nutritional (and all other) needs that were inherited from our ancestors.

Is it too late to reverse the trends that have been established. Are we too late? Are the Obstacles too great?

A major problem in answering these kinds of questions is the changes that we've made have come about too quickly (in terms of ALL our time on earth) and the safety measures that have been built into the system (the ability of the earth to repair itself) were not set up for such drastic changes. Also, as a species here on earth, there is no equal to the all-encompassing damage that our little hands have gotten us into. It's not just that WE have affected ourselves, but that our bad decisions have helped to affect ALL LIFE on this planet. We have in, a few short centuries,managed to endanger the earth itself and disrupt the ecological balance of the entire natural order.

Recently, when it was discovered that the Ozone Layer (our protection against the damaging ultraviolet rays of the sun) was being destroyed by the wanton dumping of chemicals into our atmosphere.   Can you imagine anyone with a sound mind putting profits above existence? Recently, most nations of the world got together and concluded that we need to do something to correct our environmental wrongs within the next five years or 'life as we know it, cannot continue'.   THE NEXT DAY, a headline in a major newspaper concluded that it is "Not Economically Feasible" for us to clean the environment before TWENTY years has elapsed.

In other words, business has decided that it's more important to make a profit than to survive.
It is this kind of thinking that needs to be DIRECTLY and SWIFTLY dealt with.

If we CAN return to Common Sense, then (to answer the above questions) we will survive and the goals of Health, Long Life and Happiness can be ours.

CHAPTER FOUR

THE PEOPLE OF HUNZA: LIVING LEGENDS OF LONGEVITY

Even within our own culture, there still can be found a rare individual (or even group) who has allowed their inner voice to guide them in terms of health and nutrition. These people are like small, relatively unpolluted islands in the sea of modern pollution. These brave few are using for role models those isolated places in the world today where people live somewhat close to the idyllic lifestyle of our prehistoric ancestors. In these legendary communities, the one "special" commodity that is possessed by all, is the blessing of extraordinary health. Due to a set of circumstances (that we will elaborate upon in a moment) each person in these 'special communities' EXPECTS to have a tremendously long life span, and to remain vigorous (doing hard, daily physical labor) and alert (keeping all mental and sexual powers, in tact) until very advanced years. Except for those few persons in our society who scorn the modern lifestyle and try to follow the patterns of these 'special communities', most of those in this country see these people as mere legends.

The tendency, today, is to be so skeptical and disbelieving of good health that we deny that it exists, even in others. That has been the case with all of these communities. Every year scholarly people set out on 'fact finding expeditions' to prove that the claims about these special communities are false. If they are honest, they usually return amazed at what they discover. Sometimes, however they return to the modern world with new proof that claims of longevity and health are a hoax. Here is what WE'VE determined.

Most researchers have not taken the time to examine information from the **TOTAL PICTURE**. Each investigator looks into the claims of health with a preconception about what he or she is going to find. Usually, as we've said, they go looking to dispute the claims. That is a very wrong approach. What we do is look at the total body of evidence and then consult the Inner Voice. Our conclusions are, therefore, **more** complete we feel.

Whatever 'special community' one might be examining, there seems to be some very striking similarities. These similarities appear TOO striking to be coincidental, in our opinion. As strange as it may seem to the adherents of Modern Day Advanced Technology, such 'Legendary' places in the world have but two very important similarities. Each of these communities are in very remote areas (usually mountainous valleys) and are far removed from modern, scientific advancements. Most, in fact are considered to be "living in the past", a primitive and backward life.

Secondly, the people in these special communities live happily as integral parts of nature. They do NOT see themselves as DOMINANT over their environment, but rather a flowing part of the harmonious process of life. Consequently, their diets consist mostly of wholesome, organically grown fruits, vegetables, grains and nuts. There is ordinarily an absence of good pasture land and this, in addition to a poor financial situation (by modern economic standards) prohibits any sort of animal husbandry. As another result of the 'situation' then, meat is almost never consumed and dairy products are limited to a very small amount of cheese (usually from goats).

There are four places in the world that have received the most amount of scrutiny (and therefore have stimulated the greatest controversy) on the subject of Super Health. These include 1) a valley in **Vilcabamba** (in the high regions of Ecuador ,2) **Pitcarin Island** (famous as the South Pacific landing place of the mutineers from the sailing ship Bounty), 3) The **Caucasus mountain region** in the Soviet Union, and 4) **Hunza** (with some qualifications between past and present) a community in Pakistan that is the main subject

WHERE IS HUNZA?
(And Why Are We Saying All These Great Things About It?)

The land of Hunza is located in the Karakorum Range, in the Pakistani controlled area of Kashmir. At first glance this statement may seem to be (not only confusing but) totally unimportant to our discussion. It isn't.

In fact, Hunza is in a very important strategic location for Pakistan . You see, the high peaks of the Karakorums guard the crossroads of India, Afghanistan, China, and the Soviet Union.

Unlike the Pitcarin Island population, Hunza is a good test area for health practices because of its relative size (Pitcarin has only about 100 people, while Hunza's populations hovers around 60,000).

The Hunzakuts, as Hunza's people are called, are mostly members of the Ismaelie sect of Moslems. In other words,they are a people who have God as a central part of their lives.

Even though Hunza lies at the crossroads of many important civilizations, it is made up of many extremely remote villages. This is one reason why it has remained a separate and 'in tact' society. To illustrate how remote these villages really are, the Hunzakuts' language (Burushaski) has no relationship to any other known form in the world. There is also no written form of this language and, consequently, no written history of Hunza (written by Hunzakuts) exists. All that we know about Hunza, before interference from the 'outside world', has been passed down by word-of-mouth from one generation to the next.

Some might say that this is an extraordinarily poor way to retain information within a culture, but research has shown that (because 'remembering' is taken as an important job in societies with oral traditions) the records have a tendency to be extremely accurate and almost 'word for word from one generation to the next. Most of you may remember the famous television docudrama ROOTS which based the search of the real-life character (Arthur Haley Jr.) for the African village where his great-great grandfather was captured as an American Slave, on the oral history handed down to him by his parents. When Mr. Haley went to Africa and talked to the village historian of a Mandingo tribe, the words of the village historian were 'almost exactly the same' as the ones used by his parents. So, we must conclude that this type of tradition is valid AND accurate.

Regardless of what observation method we use, there are certain things about Hunza that anyone can see for themselves. These are the inarguable truths.

Producing food in Hunza is not an easy task. This is a mountainous land, nothing is flat, therefore farming is a tricky and difficult affair. To solve this problem, the social structure of Hunza is one of sparse concentrations of people. The villages are widely separated. And the farms of Hunzaland are built on terraces cut into the hillside and built on masses of gravel which are cone or fan shaped. This design is world famous for its ingenuity and effectiveness. Because, no one area borders any other too closely, no one farm infringes on the farmland of another. Until recently, this structure was sufficient to assure an adequate supply of food for each person. But, in an ever changing world, with an ever increasing population, the ratio of workable farmland to people is becoming too small to comfortably supply the Hunzakuts with food.

This is just one of the pressures that Hunza people are dealing with. Luckily, their 'old ways' and customs are helping too relieve them of some pressures. This is because of a unique way that the people of Hunza have of governing themselves.

Until 1976 the Hunza state was ruled in a unique way, by the late Mir (ruler), Mohammad Jamal Khan. For, although the Mir had total control over both life and death in the region, the Land of Hunza was considered to be extremely democratic. The reason for this is that the Mir never used his ultimate authority without first consulting a committee of the wise and elderly (the two words were almost synonymous with one another). It was (and still is) the function of this group of respected elders to settle any problems or disputes.

Within the structure of this committee, the Mir acted as an advisor, holding daily court with the other members to resolve the problems that were presented to them. The council would sit in the open air, on carpets spread in front of the Mir's wooden throne, listening to the citizens plead their cases or make suggestions.

As we've already said, the land of Hunza consisted of many small villages, so the Mir couldn't be expected to hear every case. For this reason, each village had an appointed local chief and sergeant at arms to deal with local matters (those too trivial to disturb the Mir with).

This brief description of Hunza's social structure is presented only to show that the Hunzakuts, on all levels, oppose the complications of modern life. They also hold the elderly in high regard and very few arguments are not concluded in a timely and just fashion.

Today, they have a new 38 year old Mir who is the son of the late ruler. Since its independence in 1947, Pakistan has taken control of Hunzaland and has turned the Mir into a kind of 'senator' who speaks and votes on behalf of his people in the House of Representatives. Still, however, local affairs are left in the hands of the young, university educated Mir and his wise advisors.

HUNZA'S HEALTH SITUATION TODAY

When we discuss the health of the people of Hunza, we must make a distinction between the historical (and somewhat legendary) health of the past and the longevity, and energy of the people who inhabit the region today. Also, when we say TODAY we are referring to a span of time that might encompass the last three to five decades. The reason for these (seeming) inconsistencies, is that within this relatively brief period, many changes have taken place within the Hunza society. Even the late Mir himself talked with bitterness about the progress that had slowly altered this once isolated region. Sadly, we must report that many of the old customs and ways of the Hunzakuts are fading into the past.

And, what are some of the valuable contributions of progress that have been bestowed upon Hunzaland? The list reads like the FBI's most wanted list. We've given Hunza an increasing number of foreign visitors, a modern road to help ever growing numbers of people to reach the inaccessible regions, a modern hotel in Baltit (the capital), and the conscription of Hunza people into the Pakistani army. Along with this wonderful new contact with the outside world came also an influx of modern poisons such as tobacco, sugar, white flour, and candy. Meat, in excess, is now available (especially around the tourist centers), as are dairy products and other modern conveniences.

Still, a few remote villages resist. These, hard to reach places have remained pure, simple and natural in their ways. These isolated Hunzakuts have preserved their extraordinary health standards, their endless energy, their link with Common Sense and (as a consequence) their long span of happy life.

In general, though, all Hunza natives are feeling the pressures of progress. As one of the elderly stated,"I have been following the changes that are taking place in my state, but there is noting that anyone can do. This is the untouchable part of progress, and there is no way that it can be avoided. That is progress and modernization, and we have to pay the price for it."

As wise as this man must truly be, he still doesn't realize two important things. First, he doesn't understand that we cannot simply accept what others call 'progress and modernization' as an inevitable fact of life. If he can see where the new ways are leading his people,then he knows that he has nothing to lose by speaking (and working) against 'progress'. The alternative is death, not only for a way of life that is dear to him, but for the individuals that he loves. Secondly, he should see that those of us who have already experienced Modern Life and have (by some miracle) been enlightened to the dangers of it, long for the style of life that he already has. He should understand that we are working to change the path of progress so that we might regain what he takes for granted. He might then understand what the real price he will be paying for allowing 'progress' to overtake his style of living without a fight. Perhaps it is human nature, but often we do not know what we already have, until it is gone. But, knowing the value of what we have, it is our duty to fight to keep it.

THE LEGENDARY HEALTH AND
LONGEVITY OF THE PAST

The fact remains, even though the near perfect health of the people of Hunza is rapidly deteriorating, there is no serious problem of degenerative disease in this region (as we take for granted) and the health standards, on the whole, are much higher here than in any "modern" society. This is an indisputable fact, that has always been observed to be the case.

In fact, the famous British physician, Sir Robert McCarrison, visited Hunza at the beginning of this century and brought back amazing reports. In one of his writings, he referred to the nerves of the Hunzakuts as 'solid as cables', while, at the same time calling these wonderful people "sensitive, like a violin string." This extraordinary quality, as well as the other attributes associated with their amazing health he relates to their diet that consisted largely of fruits, grains, vegetables, nuts and green leaves.

Other researchers and visitors to the region have noted similar characteristics and have arrived at the same, or similar kinds of conclusions as to the source of these people's amazing health and longevity. But no one has a complete analysis of the elements behind their supreme health and long life. We will discuss these elements in complete detail, in a later chapter. Here, let us emphasize that, while the Hunzakuts are, today free from major degenerative diseases and live long happy lives, they were once **free from ALL disease** (both major and minor). They simply would NOT become sick. In 1958, the late Mir is quoted to have told some visitors, "Our people, young and old do not know what fatigue is." As an example of this, it has been noted that an average Hunza man of 80 or ninety years, can walk to Gilgit (a town, 65 miles from Hunza) and, on the same day, return, carrying a heavy load and immediately resume his regular daily routine of extensive hard work.   The fact is that each day for every Hunza person consists of much walking and climbing, just to 'get to work' so to speak. Remember, farmlands are sometimes quite difficult to get to.

Many books and articles have been written on this subject and substantiate this fact, with praise for the health, energy and vitality of these people. However, a few articles have recently indicated that the praises are exaggerated. What these articles do not consider is the recent negative effects of the advancement of technology and progress in Hunza.

It is no wonder that earlier literature on Hunza reports a much higher standard of health. It seems fairly certain to most that the earlier reports were not exaggerated, but that the high standards of health that these people once experienced are rapidly deteriorating.

It is essential to point out that the diet, life-style and the resulting health of these people is due to the circumstance of locality and NOT to a matter of choice.   Therefore, they were not aware of their exceptional and superior health qualities. Today, they are just now learning how lucky they really are, by reports from the media and the wise and elderly leaders are sadly beginning to determine that deterioration is taking place. Let's hope, for the sake of all humanity that these fine people are able to withstand the flow of modernization and preserve themselves as specimens of superior health and longevity.

Without people like the Hunzakuts for us to observe and speculate about, the rest of us will not know what is possible and will not know what we are missing. Because of our innate willingness to 'go along with the way things are', we need a people such as the Hunzas as a visible health standard by which to measure our society's health and to give us a goal to shoot for.

CRIME FREE STATE
(Healthy body, healthy minds)

Before leaving the subject of the social and physical structure of Hunza, we'd like to add one final, interesting note. In addition to the lack of physical disease in this land, Hunza is also reported to be remarkably Crime Free. A recent T.V. report presented confirmation from the Mir that no serious crime of any kind has been recorded in the area for hundreds of years or as far back as any living community member could recall.

In much of the literature that deals with these people, the point has been stressed that they are extremely peaceful and acts of violence, murder and other crimes of passion are simply unknown in the region. When the Mir and his elders sit in their open air court, they settle disputes of the most congenial kind. Matters of solving murders are totally foreign to them as disease and tooth decay once were. It seems illogical (and somewhat ironic) that as these people are subjected to modernization, they have also been forced to join the Pakistani army. Trying to make professional killers out of an innately peaceful people is the ultimate perversion.

The importance of such a phenomenon is greatly emphasized by the fact that these people are not 'well off' by our modern standards. Their food resources are modest and they do not have the comfortable houses, luxury cars and other modern conveniences that we take for granted.

They are a community of people who are financially poor, with very limited resources, living in a remote and difficult area with barely enough lands to produce their foods. Yet, not only are they with crime, but they are very hard working people who are entirely happy and content with their existence. This is another demonstration of the interrelation of our physical and mental health. It also shows the undeniable effect that our individual health has on the health of the community we live in and the emotional health of human society at large.

It is no coincidence that these same characteristics apply to the other "blessed communities" of the world, such as Vilcabamba in Ecuador. For, these people are all living in the same, basic circumstances, close to nature, nourishing themselves on the same kind of natural diet. Consequently, we believe, they are also content with their lot and therefore a disease and crime free community. This once again proves the value of the popular expression, " You are what you eat."

CHAPTER FIVE

THE TEN COMMANDMENTS OF 'SUPERIOR *HUNZA* HEALTH'

Contrary to popular belief, there is no ONE ingredient that is responsible for the superior health of the people of Hunza. However, there are reasons why these people enjoy the health benefits that they do. The **phenomenon** is the result of a combination of ingredients, ten elements that work together to make up the "Hunza Health phenomenon" Before we give you these ten ingredients, we'd like to make an important point, a point that we've tried to make before. Circumstance has played a vital role in every one of the communities that are famous for their superior health. It was not an intellectual choice on the part of these people to live long, healthy lives. Chance was simply on their side. The 'luck', of these people is that they have been allowed to live the way the Creator intended.

This doesn't mean that any one of us cannot actively choose to alter the course of our own life and improve our health. On the contrary, that is exactly what we are saying you should be doing. When your lifestyle is not forced upon you because of a set of circumstances, but is rather the result of an intellectual choice, then there is never the fear that you will 'lose what you learn' because of environmental changes. When you decide to live a more healthy life, when you choose to live according to the principles that the Creator set up for you, then you will be granted all the benefits intended for mankind when we were originally placed within the Garden.

1 - AIR

Air is the first and most immediate human necessity. Under the right conditions, the human body can subsist for many days without the benefit of food or water, but deprive it of oxygen for only a few minutes and the results will be quite noticeable. The fact is, without air for an average of three to four minutes the body will die.

Now, imagine how much air passes through your lungs in a single day, a week, a year a lifetime. If this air is pure, natural, unpolluted then your lungs will be better able to do the job that it was meant to do. But, when every breath you take is 'just a little bit polluted', then you are depriving your body of a necessity that it cannot function without. It seems morbidly amusing to see daily newspaper reports on the breathable quality of our air. Do you anxiously read the daily paper to find if your local air quality will be good, or slightly polluted or definitely unhealthful?

The people of Hunza are lucky to live atop a mountain range that is tens of thousands of feet high. They are far away from industry and there are no cars to pump carbon monoxide into the atmosphere. In short, their air is completely unpolluted. It is fresh, clean and totally the opposite of that which we are forced to breathe while living in our overcrowded, highly modernized cities. This should come as no surprise to you since we're certain that you've heard more than once the local T.V. weatherman warn you about breathing. Sometimes the warnings are specifically aimed at those who already have trouble with their respiratory tracts, or the elderly, or those who like to be active in the outdoors. But, often the air is so highly poisonous that it is literally unfit for all humanity. Do these reports ever bother or anger you enough to do something about the quality of life in our world? The obvious, simple solution to the problem is to move to a place far away from the crowded cities if we want clean, fresh air.   Most of us cannot do that, however. It also will not really solve the problem (as we've seen, even Hunza is becoming affected by pollution). But, is there anything you can do to improve your own health? The next best thing to moving to a place like Hunza is to get to the mountains, the deserts, the seasides, or the large parks with lots of greenery, as often as possible. Give your body a break, let it breathe the clean, fresh air as often as is possible for you.

You could also clean, purify, refresh and revitalize (enhance the oxygen) in your home and office with another method, suggested by NASA. That is to fill your living space with plenty of plants. This is important from two aspects. First, you spend a considerable amount of time in your home. To begin with you spend about eight hours sleeping in your home which is one third of the whole day. If you are retired, you might be within your home, even more of the time. If you are working in a office, or other confined work-space, you spend most of your time indoors. Second, there are a lot of pollutants in our indoor air. These indoor pollutants are very hazardous to our health and include formaldehyde fumes that are released from carpeting and building materials and unhealthy substances like benzine and carbon monoxide cigarette smoke and many others .

Dr. Wolverton senior research scientist who heads NASA'S environmental research lab. at the John C. Stennis Space Center in Mississippi has used ordinary house plants to clear indoor air of chemical fumes and every kind of pollutants for several years now. The experiments will eventually lead to air-purifying plants being placed in the spacecraft, but the NASA scientist says that green growing things can clean up the air inside an earthbound home just as well. This extensive environmental research by NASA indicates that the best method of cleaning and purifying your indoor air is by using common green plants. In the same line of thinking NASA has come up with a new design of a small air filtration and purification unit which combines the use of green house plants and activated carbon. This small unit, by combining the house plant and the activated carbon is ten time more effective and efficient in cleaning and purifying the indoor air.

Doesn't all this remind you of the garden that we were placed in, to live according to the scriptures?

The first commandment of Hunza Health then is, "Take care of the air so that it can take care of you. We need clean, fresh air as much as possible for optimum health."

2 - PURE AND LIVE WATER

Our second most immediate need in obtaining ultimate health is water. Again, we can last much longer if deprived of food, than we can without water. A quick examination of our mineral make-up, reveals that our bodies are made up almost entirely of water. This, then, is probably **THE** most vital basic building material for our very existence.

Unfortunately, our city water, is not much cleaner than the air we are forced to breathe. Tap water, in an attempt to 'improve on nature', is highly chemicalized and fluoridated. The chemicals used in water are extremely poisonous. They have to be to counter-attack the harmful bacteria that we dump into our water supplies in the form of wastes.

So, where do we go if we want to get good, clean, natural water? A few years ago, our immediate answer would have been to drink only water from a live spring or artesian well. Unfortunately, new evidence suggests that even in very remote areas, the ground waters are becoming polluted as new and greater quantities of chemicals and unnatural substances are pumped into our atmosphere and dumped on our soils and streams. So, we must qualify our answer and say that the best source of water for human consumption is first spring water then well water **IF there are no chemical wastes running into them.** Contaminations of water supplies are becoming a common occurrence. We believe that as long as our spring and well water is polluted the best choice is to drink distilled water. Distilled water is 100% pure water and can be made through evaporation of any water.

Some whole towns and even large cities are feeling the urgency of finding better water for their inhabitants. Situations where 'Peter is Robbed to Pay Paul,' have been created throughout the country. In Los Angeles, for instance, the Southern Californians must rely on the water 'acquired' from the North. Tensions become high as threats of drought in the North increase the overall value of the water in this particular state. And, California is not the only state experiencing **this kind of problem**. It **is GLOBAL**. Even though our planet's surface is more than two thirds water, we still cannot find enough CLEAN water to drink.

However, let's stay with why we think spring water is the best water for the human body. The answer to this is simple. It is the closest to the kind of water that humans have been nourished upon for millions of years. It was this kind of water that was quenching human thirst when humans were merely in the developmental stages.

Truly, it wouldn't matter if we got our water from a spring or a stream. The main concern is that it is CLEAN and UNCHANGED from its natural state. Surface water has the chance of being polluted by a number of outside sources.

Spring water USUALLY is purified in a natural way as it sinks through layers of granite and into the water-table. This is not always the case, since many modern pollutants are affecting our ground water supply directly (by seepage from waste sources). So, we must try to acquire the cleanest water (most untouched and unpolluted) available. In the deserts of Arizona I met a man and his wife who distilled all their water with an ingenious device that used sunlight and charcoal. Even though all of his neighbors drank polluted well water and worried about their situations, he was satisfied that his water was extremely clean. It was not 'directly' well water, but it was a good substitute. The point is, sometimes you cannot get the ultimate then you must do the best with what you have, and the 'best' is often very good. We believe under the present highly polluted situation the distilled water is the best choice.

In Hunza, in fact, the only water that is available is that which roars down the sides of snow covered mountains. This is NOT spring water, but as it is relatively unpolluted it is live, fresh and mineral rich. The Hunzakuts,obviously also use this water to feed the vegetables and fruits in their gardens. The special quality of living freshness, therefore is contributed to all the things that the Hunza people ingest.

In other words, the people breathe clean air and drink clean water and EAT FOODS that are nourished on clean air and water. It is no wonder they are healthy, because they adhere to the first and the second commandment of superior health. The Second Commandment being, "Thou shalt care for the water of the earth so that you can drink fresh, clean, living water and all the living things in your care can drink this water too."

3- WHOLESOME HUMAN NATURAL FOOD

While it may be true that humans cannot live for more than a few minutes without air, and only a short time if deprived of water, the most important deciding factor in human health is food. The human body is just like a complex machine that has been developing on and improving its systems with the aid of specific fuels (foods) for millions of years. Simply speaking, we **NEED** certain fuel. We were MADE to operate on certain, specific foods.

The difference between proper and improper nutrition for the body is like the difference between kerosene and "super, unleaded gasoline" for your car. Some cars might even be able to run on kerosene for a short time, but eventually (sooner than you would have if properly fueled) the engine of your car is going to quit.

Because of the importance of understanding this point, we will be devoting coming chapters to the logical, scientific explanation of exactly the kind of food that is proper for the human body.

Here, we will be outlining the specific diet of the people of Hunza, which we will be using as a guide for a balanced, natural and healthy diet. Keep in mind that their basic diet is perfectly in accordance with what we conclude to be the proper (natural) human fuel (food). It is also important to note that those other places that are also famous for their superior health and longevity (Vilcabamba etc.) have had their diet conditioned along the same dietary principles .

So, what foods do the people of Hunza eat and not eat? Since they lack good pasture land, there are few animals in Hunza, so they do not rely of them for meat or for dairy products. Also, since they are Moslems, pork is not even considered for consumption. Grains play an important role in their diets. The seasons are short in Hunza and they are forced to utilize grains wisely, saving a portion of each year's harvest for next year's planting. For this reason, poultry and, therefore eggs, are scarce, since they do not have enough excess grains to feed the chickens or other birds.

Again, due to natural circumstance (rocky hills) the most often kept animal is the goat. From this the milk is used, either to drink or in the limited production of cheese and very little butter. As we will discuss later, of all the four legged creature's milk, Goat Milk appears to be one of the closest to that of human milk. In all cases though, the primitive style of living does not allow for any chemical additives or processing that harms the natural nutrition of these foods. Also, as far as animal fat is concerned, there is none used by these people. There is virtually no frying of foods and the fat content of even prepared meals is extremely low (almost non-existent) by modern standards. The only oil that they use is obtained from the apricot seed.

What the Hunzakuts thrive on, mostly, is the famous Hunza Bread. This is made from a coarse, whole grain, barley flour and water and formed into a kind of pancake. Remember, this is **WHOLE GRAIN**, hand-ground and fresh from a clean highly fertile land.

In addition, they also eat a lot of vegetables, green leaves, fruits, grain and some nuts. Their grain selection includes wheat, barley, buckwheat, corn, millet, alfalfa, and rye. Their vegetables are mostly potatoes, tomatoes, carrots, onions, garlic, peas, beans and pulses. The fruits that are generally available in the region are mulberries, apricots, apples, cucumbers, grapes, peaches, cherries and some melons. It's an excellent variety that appears to supply all essential vitamins in precise quantities.

The diet of these people was studied by Pakistani nutritionist, Dr. S. Maqsood. He found the average caloric intake of the Hunzakuts to be about 1900 (about 2/3 that of an average American). 98 1/2% of this consisted of protein, fat and carbohydrates "from vegetable sources." The food originating in animal flesh or from dairy products comprised only about 1 1/2% of their total food intake. And, this amount is calculated from an average consumption. That means that the animal by-products part of the diet is not consistent, but rather sporadic causing little continual damage.

The most important single observation to be made about food consumption in Hunzaland is that **almost everything is eaten raw**, uncooked, just as nature intended. This preference for live food includes every kind of sprout (one of the most 'living' sources of nutrition known).

In summary then, the people of Hunza eat almost nothing in the way of meat, dairy products, eggs, animal fats or processed and chemicalized foods. The only exceptions to this come with what is now being brought into the area from the outside, as "progress" makes its unhealthy advance on the people of this peaceful mountain region. What we have outlined here appears to be the latest craze in 'healthy diets' in the U.S. , but, in fact is the classic "Hunza Health Recipe."   Our third Health Commandment then is based upon the knowledge that a community (which exists today) is surviving in a much more healthy way because they have followed (more closely) the diet that the Creator intended for us. The Commandment is this, "Work in harmony with your earth so that it will yield foods for you that consists mainly of live, organically grown grains, seeds, vegetables and nuts. Eat these raw and untampered with. The way they are given to you."

3 "A"- THE LAND

Before leaving our explanation of Health Commandment #3, there is one very important factor that must be considered. It is so important that, for emphasis we thought it would be proper to mark it separately under its own heading.

The fact is this: the land we live on, and the soil which grows our food is the original source of any life on this planet. The earth (which is another name used for land and soil) is truly the "mother of us all".

If we look at scripture we will see the direct relationship of life and earth. God created the Earth on the first day then.......... Lord God formed man from the dust of the ground............ then The Lord God made trees spring from the ground.......... . Clearly this shows that everything comes from the Land (soil, ground or earth).

Science, today also, agrees that land is the prime source of all life on earth and confirms that the most important factor in producing a highly nutritional food is the quality of the soil where the food is produced.

We would like to quote from Dr. William A. Albrecht, who is considered an expert on soil and was with the University of Missouri, Department of Soil (an interesting department to be from). He is here quoted from the Agricultural Leader's Digest, June '53: "It is high time to realize that our national health lies in our soil, and the guarantee against failing health lies in the wise management of the soil for production of nutritious foods. Fertile soils are the first requisites if we are to be well fed and healthy and, therefore, to remain a strong nation".

Another evidence which supports the importance of the quality of the soil is presented here in a quote from the famous British physician, Sir Robert McCarrison. Dr. McCarrison was stationed in Gilgit (Hunza region) and did a lot of research on the people of Hunza involving their health and longevity. "In India, the same grain, when grown on the same soil and watered in the same way, was of higher nutritive value when the soil had been manured with natural farmyard manure than when manured with artificial chemical manure".

Not only are all the ingredients of super healthy communities including Hunza and Vilcabamba organically grown under the most perfect of natural conditions, but the people of these regions improve the soil with natural compost or manure which is produced, obviously, under these same 'ideal' circumstances. Also, the water from the nearby glaciers (which supply the fields) runs over the hills and through the ravines, which are also composed of rich, black soil. As a result, the water carries a highly potent, rich mineral sediment to the farmlands which contributes even further to the luxurious and highly nutritional plant growth.

There can be no comparison between the nutritional values of produce from the fertile land of super-healthy communities and others grown anywhere in the western world.

But what is the problem with our land?

Let us tell you the secret of a fertile soil. Hidden in all soil are millions of live micro-organisms which thrive on the soil, and the decomposing matter. These tiny organisms, as a by-product of their activities produce highly rich, natural fertilizer which is in turn used by the local vegetation.

There are many modern influences, such as chemical fertilizers, pesticides and finally, acid rain that kill these micro-organisms and therefore deprive our vegetation of the benefits of natural fertilizer that would have been produced by these micro-organisms.

This chemicalization has been forced on our land for many decades. It is the main reason why our produce and fruit not only have no or very little nutritional, value but do not even have the taste or the very pleasant smell of real natural, organically grown produce.

Here we would like to take this opportunity and send a message to all those so call "Scientists" who (for personal gain) want to make us to believe that they are improving the quality of natural life.

"Dear Scientist,

You will do nothing but ruin our land, the prime source of life, by continuing with your current policies. Our Creator does not need you or your improvements. It is wrong for anyone to try to improve on His perfect work. "

This is a message that any true scientist will confirm whole -heartedly.

4 - AN ABUNDANCE OF EXERCISE

The kind of Superior Health that has been achieved in Hunza is wrought with continuous, hard, physical labor. But, contrary to what might be first thought, this is precisely the fourth requirement for a natural, healthy and long life.

In Hunza, the whole community, as part of their daily routine is engaged in a great deal of physical activity. Men work alongside their wives; young stand side by side with old. All put in long hours of toil in the orchards, gardens, and fields seemingly without any care or concern for physical tiredness. Incredibly, this work is accomplished without any aid of modern farming equipment.

And, in addition to work, these people living in such a mountainous area, are forced to hike many miles daily which compounds and adds to the amount of physical energy required of them. This rigorous daily schedule is about the same for the elderly and the very young alike, and includes all the hard physical labors for each group that uncomplicated, primitive life thrives upon. In other words, no one gets any special treatment, but then, no one really NEEDS any special treatment.

It is a known fact that, historically, humans have been a very active species. We know, by observing our 'closely related species ' (apes) and by studying primitive tribes as well as communities such as Hunza that it is the most natural thing for humans to move and work throughout the day, to keep themselves fed and for the sheer enjoyment of activity. The human body has been conditioned to a lot of physical activity for many millions of years. Securing food, defending himself against other creatures and building shelters required a great deal of "bare handed labor" to achieve success. It is also in man's 'inner nature' to be curious and try new things. That is one of true beauties of being human.

Modern technology has relieved mankind of the privilege of taking care of himself (and of challenging his mind) and has replaced that privilege with laziness. An average man today spends most of his time sitting in his armchair at his house, in a car seat, or at his job. Ironically, science actually boasts that you can sit in a chair, push a few buttons and control production of heavy machinery as it operates around you. A DOUBLE irony is that the result of this modern, "advanced" lifestyle is a number of ailments such as fatigue, and the worst of all, OBESITY. For this reason, exercise has become an alternative to actual work.

If you are not blessed with a regular job that includes a good deal of physical work, you should be doing daily exercise. Good healthy exercise could also mean that you involve yourself in activities like farming, gardening, hoeing, planting, walking, climbing or carrying, or some sort of equivalent work.

The only thing you should not be afraid of when you exercise is overdoing it. You cannot exercise too much. The more you do (and are ABLE to do comfortably), the better off you'll be. As general rules, you should first choose a type of exercise that you enjoy and regardless of your age, light work for long durations is better than short periods of heavy work. In fact, you should try to avoid heavy exercise like weight lifting, wrestling and the like.

As a caution, if you haven't been doing physical work or exercise for a long period of time (and have been eating conventional foods) it might be wise to have a check-up to analyze your present health condition before starting any exercise. In any event, when you do begin to exercise, start slowly, with the minimum amount of time and increase gradually for the best results. We also recommend exercise highly which stresses NATURAL body movement. Running, walking, swimming, climbing or sports that contain elements of these will stir the 'ancient human' within you, as they are activities that have been delighting humans for millions of years. Remember too, if you've been eating conventional foods for a long time in addition to avoiding exercise, then the statement "no exercise is enough" does not apply to you. You may hurt yourself if you try to make your body do more than inferior fuels (foods) are capable of allowing. All health requirements are related to one another, just as we are related to the total creation. The Fourth Health Commandment then is, "Let your body move, naturally."

5- ADEQUATE SLEEP

A peaceful sleep is one of the important ingredients of "Hunza Health." Sleep time is when your body should be resting in a supremely relaxed state . In this way each cell will be getting revitalized and ready for another day of hard work. Our only recommendation is that you give your body as much sleep time as it requires. You will be surprised to learn that as you change to natural human food and observe the other Hunza Health Commandments (especially exercise) your sleep time will become much more restful and the need for it will decrease. New information points to the conclusion that about six hours of sleep is enough for most people, even those in the most ordinary of health in our modern society.

After a reasonable amount of time adhering to the principles of the Health Commandments, you will experience new dimension in sleeping. It will become so restful and deep that you could not have before, imagined it.

As for a recommendation on the time to sleep, we refer to the old adage, "early to bed and early to rise, makes a man healthy, wealthy and wise." Seeing the sun rise and set, experiencing the beauty of the day and the natural restfulness of the night will help you to keep in better tune with the ebb and flow of creation's natural time schedule.

Our Fifth Commandment for Hunza Health? "Thou shalt get as much sleep as YOUR BODY TELLS YOU THAT YOU NEED."

6 - MODERATE SUNSHINE

Sunshine is the only source of natural energy for every living thing upon this earth. All life - plant or animal, in the water or on the land, needs the energy of the sun. In a way, an argument could be made that ALL life on earth is merely a FORM of the sun's energy.

The human body is a part of life and also needs this energy. The sun supplies our bodies with a number of valuable nutritional elements in the form of vitamins. The latest evidence points out that emotional happiness is linked to sunlight. People who are deprived of sunlight are more depressed than those who get their fair share. It has also been recently proven that the amount of sun that you receive (through your eyes) determines how well you sleep at night. Those people who do not get out into the sun, or those who have adopted the unnatural life-style of staying up all night and sleeping during the day will not sleep as soundly (or benefit from sleep as much) as those who keep a more natural routine.

A problem has developed in recent years whereas sunshine has become harmful to us (due to pollution) instead of being beneficial as nature had intended. It's maddening to know that, due to our own stupidity we can no longer go into the sunshine, feeling the soothing warmth upon our faces, without fearing skin cancer. Our so called 'leaders' are not any help, since their only concerns are to promote business and the economy. What do we do when elected officials suggest that, to counteract the lessening of the Ozone layer, we all go around wearing hats? Don't these people understand that while WE can wear hats the rest of creation cannot? Should we start making hats for the plants and animals? The plankton in the ocean? The birds of the air? The sea creatures?

We USED to tell our readers that,"Whenever you can give your body moderate sunshine, you will be giving it a valuable source of energy." Now, again we must modify even this simple axiom.   The people of Hunza enjoy a lot of sunshine the year round. And, so far, skin cancer is not a problem for them. In that case, our 6th Commandment of Health is, "Get daily, moderate amounts of sunshine. But you must be warned that too much sunshine can create health problems". If you are burning, or other discomforts develop then you are getting too much. Continued discomfort might indicate that you need professional attention.

7 - FASTING AND RELAXATION

In Hunza there is very little land that is fit for cultivation. Consequently, there is barely enough food for the gradually overpopulating community. There are times when there is little or no food available to any family. Usually, once a year in late Spring and a few days before they begin to harvest the new crops, they will run out of food. During such periods the people go on a compulsory fast. This is the time when their digestive tracts are given a rest and their bodies a chance to cleanse themselves.

As a law of nature, when food is not sustained within the system, the body will start to use its reserve energy by first burning the extra fat cells and then gradually the old and ill cells, converting these to energy.

In a society like ours which has become addicted to overeating, a revolutionary but effective method for cleansing the body (especially the digestive system) is fasting. This will also give your body the opportunity to burn away ill, old and fat cells. There are many different methods for fasting. To name but a few, we must include Water Fasting, Wheat Grass Fasting, and Fruit Juice Fasting.

In this book we will not be going into the subject of fasting to any length. The reasoning behind the method, the various ways to fast, the experiments that have been done and the results that have been achieved by this method could be topics for a lengthy book all by themselves. We will be talking in generalities here, telling you that some fasting methods are quite beneficial and that dramatic results of curing a variety of diseases have been achieved by these methods.

There are many books on the subject of Fasting and it is scheduled to be the topic of one of our own, future publications. It should be mentioned, however, that fasting is a rapid method for cleansing the body of accumulated, toxic material, and it is in tune with the laws of nature. It has been commonly observed that animals avoid eating when they don't feel completely healthy.

In the wild, also, animals are observed to be 'at their very best' when they are hungry. Nature has provided, for instance, that when an animal is hungry (we mean

TRULY hungry in this case) all senses and reactions are sharpest. Naturally, when an animal is well fed, it is sluggish and relaxed. Even the lion or tiger in the jungle is a relatively peaceful creature unless motivated by hunger.

We should also point out that the people in "traditional" places like Hunza or Vilcabamba, do not NEED to fast, as generation to generation they have been enjoying toxic-free food, air and water. It is only people of modern and advanced societies, or people like those in Hunza who have begun to change their ways (which apparently some have) who are accumulating toxic wastes and , therefore, must resort to such measures. On the other hand, to go without food for periods of time (up to and more than 24 hours) is very common. These people do not even consider this a fast, but rather a part of their natural time schedule. An old Zen proverb suggests that to be enlightened is nothing more than eating when hungry and sleeping when tired. Good health, we would say, is a by-product of this same method and therefore our 7th Commandment says, "Eat only enough to satisfy your hunger. Let your body rest at other times."

8 - THE SENSE OF LOVE AND USEFULNESS

There has been two important studies in the Caucasus of the Soviet Union (another Super-healthy community called Abkhazia) that relate to how these two senses are maintained in Hunza. The first study, dealing with individuals above the age of eighty, showed that almost all of these people are married and have been for the length of their adult lives. The number of single people who are of advanced age is very small. This indicates that an important element in longevity is the mutual love and caring of a close human relationship.

Another study was conducted by Prof. Pitzkhelauri of the Soviet Union. His work was done with 15,000 elderly people who were above the age of eighty and living in the same area. The study revealed that those individuals who had lost their feeling of usefulness in the community died shortly thereafter.

These two studies are especially striking when viewed in the light of the Hunza population. There the aged enjoy a very high social status, in the community as well as in the family. Elderly people always live with family and close relatives, which often makes for an outstandingly large household. However, even in these large families the elderly are the center of attention, occupying a privileged position. The elderly are esteemed for their wisdom in Hunza, and the young universally believe that this is derived from long life and extensive experience. This makes the aged person's word as acceptable as law.

Let's contrast this treatment of the elderly with the way they are dealt with in our own society. As part of modernization and civilization, individuals are systematically disposed of when they reach retirement age. We detach an elderly man (for instance) from his work, his family, the society and dump him in one of our OLD AGE HOMES.

In Hunza, family members almost always consult the eldest member when making any major decision. This love and respect in both family and community, plus the physical and economical work that these people do helps to give the people of Hunza, well into ages over one hundred, a sense of responsibility, love and usefulness. This sense of usefulness is highly important in any individual in order for him to continue to live to these advanced ages. Psychologists have repeatedly reinforced this fact: Once a person concludes in his own mind that his existence no longer has any purpose, at that point he has verified his own Death Certificate.

In Hunza, and all their counterpart communities who are famous for superior health and longevity, there is no forced or accepted retirement age. The elderly are NOT thrown out of the family or the community and their sense of responsibility is not taken away from them, as is the case in most modern societies.

Another point should also be stressed. In a modern society, the elderly have already lost most of their physical and some of their mental faculties. In Hunza, those of advanced age (even in excess of one hundred years) are capable, physically and mentally, to continue performing their usual duties and responsibilities. In our own society, the elderly are often unable to care for themselves. What makes that difference is the topic of this book, or more exactly is the what makes up the body of the Ten Commandments Of Hunza Health. These ten elements of health are exactly the same in Hunza and its counterpart communities, while they are lacking in those societies that we call "advanced and modern."

9- LIMITED WORRY AND STRESS

Anyone would certainly agree that life in a remote, mountain valley, where peace and tranquility abound, would be a little easier to deal with than all the hassles we have in modern life. If we were lucky enough to live in a place where the air is fresh and clean, the water pure and living, the food wholesome and natural, and where we were literally hundreds of miles away from the nearest fear, worry, emotional complication or stress, we would probably want to live to be as old as possible.

On the other hand, in our modern society phrases are commonly heard that indicate an unwillingness to even live another day. "I just can't take it anymore," or "It's just too much for me," or our favorite, "life is just too hard sometimes," are all examples that modern 'ease' has something lacking for the human spirit.

If we had the time, we could list hundreds of stresses and emotional pressures that are an integral part of modern life, but are unknown in communities such as Hunza. To name but a few, there is the stress of driving in traffic, the daily stress of jobs, worries about weight (either being too fat, or the new one, being too skinny), worries about paying bills, fear of unemployment, fear of physical safety and security of property, law suits from enemies, worries about health and so on.

Surely, the people of Hunza have things that they must think about, goals and desires. But, these are limited and center around securing food, shelter and clothing, or, on the intellectual/emotional side, revolve around marriage, family and children.   It can be said that their environment, lifestyle and social structure contribute greatly to limiting their worries and promoting peace of mind. This healthy social atmosphere is another important element in supreme physical and mental health for the people of Hunza. As our model, it points the way for our Ninth Commandment of Hunza Health, which could be stated, "Thou shall appreciate EVERYDAY, the gift of life you have been given, and to this end not let your stresses and fears get the best of you."

10- LACK OF GREED AND ENVY

Greed and Envy are important factors in any modern society which bases the success of individuals according to their relative status in that society. How we measure our status, as compared to our neighbors, is not important. The issue is not whether we are capitalists or socialists, speak one language or another. When it comes to Greed and Envy the result to human health is going to be serious harm.

It's interesting, but it seems as though Greed and Envy actually work just the opposite of what logic would dictate. Logic tells us that a person who has very little will have a stronger desire to have more than a person who is relatively well off. It is also logical that we should only desire to be like others, or have what others possess IF we believe that they possess something valuable and good. On both counts,however, general practice shows us that this is not how these two negative forces work.

The thirst of Greed becomes stronger, most often, the more that one acquires. The more one gets, in other words, the more he wants. In addition, people usually end up desiring what their neighbor has, even if that thing has never meant anything to them before they knew that somebody else had it. This is true even when people know that something is harmful to them. This is the kind of thing that causes teenagers to use drugs. These kids are educated to the effects of drugs. They know that they might even DIE from using them (even once) but they do it just the same...because everyone else does. The famous 'Keeping Up With The Joneses' philosophy sums up this distorted way of thinking.

For the people of Hunza, there is very little in the way of 'earthly goods' and none of the modern conveniences that are taken for granted in an advanced society are available to them. But, they possess peace of mind.

It is amazing, at first glance that Greed, Jealousy, Envy and Hatred are totally foreign to the people who seem to have nothing, until we realize that they possess a life-style that is in harmony with nature and the Laws of the Creator.

The Tenth Commandment of Hunza Health then is one that is also featured (in a way) in the Ten Commandments of Old Testament Scripture,"Thou shall not Envy or Desire what belongs to another."

But, if one is in harmony with the natural laws, and follows the Commandments of Health, then he/she will possess health, be happy, live long and have wants and desires in accordance with these same principles.

NOTE: Some people might not like our presentation as the Ten Commandments of Health. But, if you are offended, ask your inner voice to guide you, we believe that you will see the wisdom in our presentation. These Commandments of Health SHOULD be directly associated with the Creator, because they are based upon the natural laws that He has set down for us. We should start to interpret our health habits in direct association with the Creator and His plan for us, for only in that way will our thoughts about health receive from us the respect that they deserve.

CHAPTER SIX

THE FOOD 'RECIPE' FOR HUNZA HEALTH

So far you have read about the importance of using (and trusting) your own common sense. We've shown how human food and a human diet have developed to the present stage. You have also read about how the Hunza people live and of their ten effective elements of superior health, vitality and longevity. Take a moment to ask yourself if what we've said so far is 'the truth'. If you let your inner voice guide you, we're confident that you'll now want to continue with what we call "The Hunza Health Recipe". This chapter is dedicated to the most important of the ten elements, the food.

In this section we will give you specific ways to prepare your menus in a healthful and more naturally attuned way. But, this is not really a recipe book. There are many good recipe books out there even some with good NATURAL FOODS recipes for you to try. What we hope to help you adopt, at the end of this reading, is a sensible eating pattern, which will be close, if not exactly like that which the people of Hunza are now using or (better yet) were using.

Let us clarify this one point; there is no way that we, in our modern society, could exactly adopt the eating pattern or lifestyle of these people. There are too many variables, environmental or social elements that would make that impossible. What we can do though, is gradually change the effects of the conditioning of modern society, until we have come as close to the lifestyle and eating patterns of these people (or a natural way of life) as our own set of circumstances will allow. The only way to live exactly the way the people of Hunza do is to go and live in Hunza itself. For some, that is a good option, but that doesn't mean that everyone (or even MOST of us) should try to find perfection in some other place than where we are now. For one thing, if everyone who is reading this book DID, suddenly move to Hunza, then Hunza would NOT be such a nice place to live any longer. For another thing, we don't want people to feel that health "in our own society" is an impossibility. We NEED everyone who is health conscious to STAY HERE, and help to change the ideas of our society as a whole.

For those of you who cannot move to Hunza or those who've made the brave choice to stay and help change things for the better (starting with your own body) here are some suggestions about the foods that you eat and ways to prepare them.

WHAT YOU SHOULD NOT EAT

Before we tell you what to eat, let us tell you what you should not eat. It is very important to stay away from certain foods. Actually, although these items are called foods, they are in fact nothing more than mild poisons.

We should completely abandon (either by the revolutionary or gradual method, explained in a later chapter) most conventional foods, but especially the following items: any kind of meat, including poultry and fish; any dairy products; all processed foods, either in packages or in cans; any food containing white flour, sugar, chemicals in the form of additives, preservatives, flavors, colorings, or others, any kind of alcoholic beverages, soda drinks, coffee or black tea.

We know, that if you've come this far with us, then you're aware that these things are not supplying your body with the nutritional elements it needs. In fact, most everything mentioned above can be, not only considered unhealthy, but POISONOUS.

We also know that some of those who are reading this book are saying to themselves, "So what's left? That's my entire diet!" Or, "This is a very strict and limited diet and is not possible. " If you are such a person, please do not be discouraged and don't make any final judgment. Be patient, keep on reading the book and all the material which comes with it.

WHAT TO EAT

The foods recommended in this book are a combination of high quality, natural foods, blessed with a great degree of healing qualities. The foods prepared by nature, as fit for mankind, can be grouped into five broad categories. These are **Vegetables** (Category 1), **Green Leaves** (Category 2), **Fruits** (Category 3), **Grains & Legumes** (Category 4) and **Nuts & Seeds** (Category 5). We have included a chart in this book and grouped the above under only four headings. The only difference between these headings and our five broad categories is that in our categorization we have combined the vegetables and green leaves under one heading. Please don't let this confuse you. We hope that this distinction will become clearer at the close of this chapter.

All the natural foods recommended here are extremely health giving, for any "perfectly healthy" person, but we should caution you. The people of Hunza have been eating natural foods and living healthy lifestyles for many generations. Most of us in a modern society, because of genetics or due to many years of filling our systems with polluted air, water, toxic foods and poisonous chemicals, have one or more weak or damaged organs. We aren't "perfectly healthy" as are the people of Hunza. We must, therefore expect a period of 'putting things in order' where we might experience some unusual sensations, perhaps even mild discomfort if and when we change to complete raw, live foods.

On the other hand, some of the natural foods recommended here are high in their fat or sweet content (such as avocados and dates) or are highly concentrated foods such as raisins and nuts. Therefore, the organic defects which exist in many of us may make it difficult for us to handle (or digest) such strong or concentrated items. This will vary from individual to individual and it will be up to you to determine, through personal experiment, which items effect hardship on your system. When these items are discovered you should either avoid them or use such foods as little as possible. On the positive side, it is often reported by those who change over to a natural foods diet, that after a relatively short time , such problems will go away.

However, it should also be cautioned that the early period of discomforts, which is the result of the food changeover and the body's natural cleansing process (which is completely explained in a later chapter) should not be mistaken for these kinds of organic weaknesses or for the effects of specific food items. When all else fails (or BEFORE ALL ELSE FAILS) please exercise your Common Sense and address any questions you might have to your Inner Voice. It's been made available to you, by a caring Creator, for just such emergencies.

The next few pages contain lists of natural food items, all properly prepared for human consumption, and related important notes to consider for beginning a new life of natural health.

VEGETABLES AND GREEN LEAFS
(Category 1 & 2)

Alfalfa Sprouts	Eggplant	Parsnip
Artichoke	Endive	Peas
Asparagus	Fennel	Pepper
Broccoli	Garlic	(Green & Red)
Beets	Horseradish	Potato
Brussels Sprouts	Kale	Pumpkin
Cabbages	Kohlrabi	Radish
Carrots	Lambs-quarter	Radish leafs
Cauliflower	Leaks	Rutabaga
Celery	Lettuce	Spinach
Chard	Mint	Squash
Chive	Mushrooms	Sweet potato
Corn	Mustard Greens	Tomato
Comfrey	Okra	Turnip
Dandelion	Parsley	Watercress

FRUITS   (Category 3)

Apple	Grape	Peaches
Apricot	Grapefruit	Pear
Avocado	Guavas	Persimmon
Banana	Honeydew	Pineapple
Blackberry	Kumquat	Plum
Blueberry	Lemon	Pomegranate
Boysenberry	Lime	Prune
Cantaloupe	Loquat	Quince

Cherries	Mandarin orange	Raspberry
Cranberry	Mango	Rhubarb
Currant	Melon	Strawberry
Dates	Muskmelon	Tangerine
Elderberry	Nectarine	Watermelon
Fig	Olive	Zapote
Gooseberry	Orange	

GRAINS AND LEGUMES (Category 4)

Alfalfa	Beans Pinto	Millet
Barley	Beans Red Kidney	Oats
Beans Azuki	Black-eyed pea	Rice (Brown)
Beans Black	Buck Wheat	Rye
Beans Haba	Clover	Soybean
Beans Lime	Corn	Triticale
Beans Mug	Dahl	Wheat
Beans Navy	Lentil	Garbanzo

NUTS AND SEEDS (Category 5)

Almond	Macadamia	Sesame seed
Brazil Nut	Peanut	Squash seed
Cashew	Pecan	Sunflower seed
Chestnut	Pinon	Walnut black
Flax seed	Pistachio	Walnut English
Hazelnut	Pumpkin Seed	

IMPORTANT NOTES

1 - <u>Produce</u> The best results come when the food you eat is fresh natural, raw and wherever possible, organically grown.Public uncertainty about use of chemical fertilizers and pesticides has made this term a common selling strategy. Make sure that what you buy IS, in fact, organically grown. It may **not** be. Just because the supermarket trying to get your money says so, doesn't make it true. Ask for proof. If you don't get it, shop elsewhere.

2 - <u>Dried Fruit</u> Any dried fruits, including nuts must be naturally dried. Nothing should be toasted, roasted, salted, or dried   through any process other than by the sun, and none should have any chemicals added.

3 - <u>Oil</u> Any oil of nuts and seeds can be used. The oil should be mechanically pressed (cold pressed), unrefined, unfiltered with no chemicals in the form of preservatives or additives. Olive Oil has proven itself to be the most healthful of all oils, and should be used if you have an opportunity to choose.

4-<u>Sweetening</u> For sweetening use honey, maple syrup, dates or date syrup. The honey and syrups should be pure, natural, unheated, unrefined, unfiltered and organic. Molasses is slightly better than refined sugar. It has some nutritional value, although it is really not much better than straight sugar, which it is derived from. Carob, is always better than chocolate. There is NO comparison between the two.

5 - <u>Salt</u> Stop salt completely and instead use other natural herbs, spices and/or lemon juice. The use of salt, even the pure sea salt and in little amounts makes a big difference on overall health. This is a strong addiction for many people, we understand. If you must use it, use as

little as possible and try gradually to phase it out. And, if you have to use ANY salt, use only pure sea salt and stay away from the common table salt in the supermarkets,as they are made of chemicals, and highly toxic.

6 - <u>Washing</u> All vegetables must be cleaned thoroughly in order to   wash away the possible chemical dust sprayed on them. This is merely a precaution and unnecessary in most cases, IF you **KNOW** your food is organically grown.

7 - <u>Peeling</u> Whenever possible, do not peel the vegetables or fruits such as carrots, cucumbers, apples and the like. There are people who even eat oranges with the membranes. Nature has universally made a design for the seeds of life, and that is to surround the seed (even the human seed), with valuable nutrients. The skin of fruits and vegetables usually contain MOST of the vitamins and nourishment for the seeds.

8 - <u>Grain and Legumes</u>   The best way to eat grain and legumes is to sprout them. The second to the best is to grind them and make Hammous (mostly done with legumes). The third choice is to cook it in the form of bread or cereal.
For sprouting buy wheat, barley, etc., unhulled. If you cannot find unhulled barley and other grain at your health shop, try any farm supply store, as most health shops do not have all the unhulled grain. If your grain won't sprout (which is rare), throw it away   it's dead! And, probably toxic.

9 - <u>Herb Tea</u>   Use your choice, but make sure it is a cleansing agent and it is naturally or preferably wildly grown, and unprocessed.

10 - <u>Spice</u> Use any natural dried herb and spices. Only make sure that there are no foreign materials or chemicals added. These too should be naturally dried. Buying whole, fresh herbs and drying them yourself is a fun, healthy hobby.

HOW TO PREPARE FOOD

By now, you know what you should not eat and what are the proper human food items. Here we are going to show you ways to prepare your food, if you prefer to follow conventional eating patterns while eating a natural diet. Some people take this lifestyle a step further by breaking conventional conditioning altogether and this makes life much more simple and easy for them. They just eat their food items raw, as they are, without any preparation or even mixing. This is the ideal if you can do it. But, we admit that not many people can, either due to habit, tradition or personal preferences. Very few start on the road to Hunza Health by making such a radical change and infinitely few ever evolve to that stage, so we will here show you how to stay with natural foods while remaining within conventional habits.

We are going to give you a number of general guidelines for food preparations, mixing and combining. We will leave the details of your recipes to your own imagination and tastes. There are also a great many fine, natural foods recipe books on the market that can be used. We would welcome any interesting recipes or food preparation suggestions that you have come up with. If your recipe is used in our publications, your name will appear in print. There will also be prizes awarded for the best three recipes that are presented for publication, and you will receive a complimentary copy of the publication that your recipe appears in.

Send your recipes to
Center For Human Natural Nutrition
15015 Ventura Blvd.,
Sherman Oaks, CA 9140

Now, on to the broad categories of food preparations, mixing and combining.

CATEGORY ONE
(VEGETABLES)

Vegetables are one of the most important food categories, supplying vital nutritional elements to the human body. Hundreds of different combinations of vegetable salads can be prepared. If you prefer to eat vegetables such as carrots, celery, cabbage, cauliflower, tomatoes, cucumbers or any of the rest, as the Creator gave them to us (without mixing, in other words), then by all means the sky is the limit. There are some vegetables, we've discovered that are great alone, but seem to take on a whole new taste when mixed with other vegetables.

Should you decide to Mix And Match, remember, you don't have to stick with vegetables in your salads. A little sprinkling of Hunza Bread Crumbs is far tastier and much healthier than any store-bought crouton. All of the bread recipes for the more industrious can be twisted and shaped into tiny 'noodles' as well. A cool, pasta salad on a hot summer day is a sure favorite.

There are a number of fine books out on the subject of salad AND dressing preparation. The most common, natural food dressings are made by mixing oils (mostly olive oil, or other cold pressed oils, as specified in the Important Notes To Human Natural Food Items section) with fresh lemon or lime juice, a touch of honey and a number of natural herbs and spices. Another commonly used recipe is one using ripe avocado, blended with the oil of your choice and then adding lemon juice and any other item you like.

CATEGORY TWO
(GREEN LEAVES)

The four categories of basic food items, vegetables, fruits, grains & legumes, and nuts & seeds are well known to the American people. But, a fifth category, green leaves is not very well known as an important food item to many people in America, even today.

In advanced countries, until very recently, green leaves were considered little more than animal food. Some 'refined' individuals thought that to eat vegetables and especially green leaves was merely a sign of poor economic status. This perspective, again, couldn't be further from reality.

All recent nutritional research proves that green leafy foods are essential for the healthy maintenance of the human machine. Interestingly, in modern countries, the most commonly consumed Raw Vegetable is lettuce, which (in dinner salad) is seen by restaurant owners as a "cheap way to fill up the customers" while most home-makers find it an easy (inexpensive) substitute for Real Vegetables. What is amusing is that in our chemicalized society, the lettuce leaf has become almost non-nutritional. When tested recently against almost all other vegetables, common table lettuce ranked at or near ZERO on all counts except being a source of roughage.

In most communities that are not so 'advanced' as we are, a lot of green leaves, in their natural, live state are consumed. As a result, many of the diseases and 'health complications' (such as constipation and colon problems) that we hear so much about in modern society are unheard of in the, so called 'primitive' cultures.

Green leaves that you should consider for your own diet (if you are not already using them regularly) are spinach, kale, radish leaves, watercress, mint, parsley, alfalfa sprouts and others. How should you eat them, and in what quantities? A good portion could be from three to five ounces of any one or a combination of your favorites. Let your natural instincts (as was discussed earlier in the Commandments section) be your guide. When you determine that natural hunger needs to be satisfied, then here are some points to consider:

1. Eat your green leaves as the Creator gave them to you. Raw leaves are best. You can also chop and mix them with raw vegetables to create unique tastes with or without oil and/or lemon juice etc.

2. They can be chopped and mixed with your usual salad items. Years ago, most of us at the Center thought that salads were lettuce, tomatoes and carrots (and that's all). Now, when discussing the topic amongst ourselves, we're interested to find that just about every kind of raw vegetable and green leaf finds its way into our salad bowls.

3. They can be sliced or chopped and rolled into your Hunza Bread to be eaten like natural Hot Dogs.
Remember, chop your green leaves 'just before' using them. Do not keep them, as they lose their potency with age.

CATEGORY THREE
(FRUITS)

We have been conditioned to think of fruit as something other than REAL food for some reason. It is most commonly seen as a 'snack' that is healthier than candy and cookies. In a modern, advanced society such as ours fruits are viewed somewhat like 'desserts of non-preference.' That means that they are the kind of dessert we are supposed to eat when something else that is REALLY GOOD is not available.

We've been conditioned to see the sweets,cakes, candies, ice creams and other devitalized and toxic foods as the REAL treats, while fruits have taken on a role as a 'half food'.

The truth of the matter is, by the laws of nature and human physiology, fruits are a complete human food and thus are extremely important for the maintenance of vibrant health. They are the perfect food for modern humans in our opinion since fruits are not only handy, self contained in most cases, but can be utilized in a number of ways. They are universally SWEET as well, and sometimes it's better to give into habits (such as a sweet tooth) in as healthy a way as possible rather than to give UP on health.

Here are some ways you might like to try fruits:

1. Separately, as the Creator gave them to us. They are especially good if you can get them fresh off the tree or bush. Buying a few trees or shrubs for your yard, or even a book about wild fruits might be good investments that will enhance your life (and even lengthen it).

2. By mixing them into a fruit salad you can have all the benefits that were addressed in the Vegetable Salad section. You might also want to try mixing your fruits and vegetables for a spring salad that defies description.

3. In the form of ICE CREAM fruits can supply you with your nutritional needs AND satisfy the child in all of us. This method of utilization is also a sure favorite with REAL children. To accomplish this special recipe, place

a combination of your favorite FRESH fruits into your freezer for 12 to 24 hours. When they are good and frozen, grind the mixed, frozen fruits through a meat grinder or other grinding machine. The results are largely a result of trial and error, depending upon the right combination of fruits to suit your tastes. What you'll get is an ice-cream-like substance without the cream or calories. You can add honey for extra sweetness, or carob powder and any other natural toppings that you prefer.

CATEGORY FOUR
(Grains And Legumes)

Grains and legumes are the most important food category in the whole world. This category supplies the bulk of the all real nutrition to underdeveloped countries. These food items offer the most effective source of roughage (fiber) and a host of nutritional elements.

All grains and legumes can be used in three different ways. You can sprout them and eat them as a true living food, or make bread or other things from the sprouts. You can also grind them to flour and make bread and cake or mix the flour with oil and make something like hammous (the name of a Middle East recipe, which we will explain later) from the mix. The third way is simply to cook them and eat them that way.

A-- Breads and Cakes

There are many varieties of breads that you can prepare and this is good. Bread is a major food staple for the people of Hunza, therefore it seems like a good idea for us to eat a lot of it too. But, please don't go out and spend lots of money on prepackaged products. When we are talking about bread, we have certain principles and characteristics in mind.

1. Your basic ingredients should all be 100% stone ground, whole wheat (or other whole grain) flour. Water should be as clean and fresh as possible and when using salt, use only evaporated sea salt. If, occasionally, bran can be added to your recipes, it will prove extremely valuable in supplying more roughage and fiber for your body to cleanse itself with.

2. Breads and cakes can be molded into a number of different shapes by using a variety of mixtures. That, in our opinion is one of the beauties of them. We can eat something different every night and still be eating basically the same, healthful ingredients.
For instance, bread is commonly made into loaf forms. If this is your preference, then natural yeast is a must. Otherwise, you can produce your breads in small, pancake like shapes. Some of our more industrious customers have said that they like to bake their breads, like cookies, in animals shapes for their children. For sweetening, if desired, you can mix and combine ingredients such as honey, dates, raisins, other dried fruits, molasses (use sparingly), and various chopped nuts. {There's a great idea for Hunza Pizza, later in this chapter.}

3. The Hunza Method Bread: Blend the flour with salt (1/2 tsp. of salt for every two cups of flour) and add enough water to knead it on a lightly floured surface to prevent sticking. Knead until you have a very stiff consistency of dough, cover it with a wet cloth and leave it at room temperature for about one or two hours. At the end of that time, take the dough and shape small round balls (about 1 1/2 to 2 inches in diameter) and roll them on a lightly floured surface until you have a stack of

pancake-like breads, about 10 to 12 inches across. For a natural yeast, keep one of the balls of dough under the wet cloth for 24 hours and mix it with your next day's batch of dough.

4. Cooking: The best method for cooking is to form the pancake like bread and NOT COOK IT AT ALL. Simply leave your formed cakes out in the sun, or in an oven with a temperature of UNDER 130 degrees. Another method is to leave the oven set low and THE DOOR OPEN. This will prevent the bread from cooking too fast, which destroys the nutritional value of the living grains.
If you feel you MUST cook then, the second best method is to follow the recipe above and the procedures suggested, then cook at a normal baking temperature.

B-- SPROUTS

Sprouts from grains and legumes such as alfalfa, wheat, barely, triticale, buckwheat, lentil and many other beans and seeds are LIVE FOODS of the highest nutritional value. That is because they are LIVING FOOD, still alive, in fact, when we eat them. Therefore, they are programed with all the building blocks of life.
When preparing your own menus of High Quality Natural Foods, please try and include generous portions of sprouts in your diet, especially of grains and alfalfa. You can make no single, better choice as an addition to your current diet.

1. How To Use Sprouts: Sprouts can be added to any vegetable salad and will greatly enhance the nutritional value as well as the taste of the mixture. Sprouts can also be eaten "as is". One of our favorite 'all sprout' recipes is to mix wheat, barely and triticale sprouts. Sometimes a

Sometimes a sprinkling of olive oil, lemon juice, honey or other natural herbs and spices creates an even more exciting snack.

2. <u>Grinding Sprouts:</u> The full nutritional value of sprouts can be retained, while changing the texture, by grinding the sprouts into a paste and adding natural flavors. For a sweet taste, add honey, maple syrup, nuts and spices like cinnamon. For something unique try a combination of lemon juice (or other juices), oils, onion powder, garlic, or a variety of spices can only serve to increase your love of sprouts. Be experimental, sprouts are also cheap especially if you grow them at home. If you come up with a combination that doesn't suit you, you haven't lost much. If, on the other hand, you discover a true taste treat, then all the better! Another good reason to grow your own sprouts is, obviously, you won't have to worry about the grocer spraying chemicals on your living foods.

One more thing, your ground sprouts can be added to just about any recipe, by the way. We like the paste spread on Hunza Bread, like butter.

3. <u>Making Sprout 'Bread':</u> Here's a neat trick, you can also grind sprouts and knead the paste into a stiff dough! Adjust the thickness of the dough, by adding small amounts of 100% stone ground whole wheat (or your favorite) flour, and small amounts of water. A little water makes your dough thinner, and a little flour does the opposite. When you get the consistency you desire, the dough can be used in the same way as was explained for bread and cake. As with breads and cakes, your own imagination is your only limitation in preparing the sprout-dough in a variety of shapes, sizes and recipes.

C--HAMMOUS

As mentioned, one of the ways to eat the legumes is to grind them (soak in water for 24 hours for easy grinding) and mix the result with oil (we usually recommend olive oil--but use other oil if you don't like olive oil) and then add spices (garlic for sure) and some fresh lemon juice. This makes a delicious food when you eat it with bread. In Middle Eastern recipes, Garbanzo beans are most often used to make a delicious Hammous dish. But, again, you can try any other beans that you like.

CATEGORY FIVE
(NUTS AND SEEDS)

There is another natural food that has somehow gotten confused in our nutritional thinking, from the time we were developing into our present state. These often maligned, wholly natural foods are nuts. Some people will tell you that nuts are merely items that they eat IN ADDITION to their foods. Others call them "bird seed". This is a twisted perspective. Nuts are a highly concentrated, nourishing and natural food item. In nature, we once thrived on almost nothing else. How can you enjoy them?

1. As the Creator gave them to us. One good thing about nuts, we've found, is that they take time and effort to eat. This is good. Our natural ancestors had to do a little work to get their foods. We probably will benefit by doing the same with ours. Because of the effort involved in each tasty nut, you cannot gorge yourself on them as with other foods. Depending upon the nuts (or seeds) chosen, it might take dozens to get a mouthful. These are favorites for those of us who need to do a little dieting. When you eat nuts for an hour or so, you feel like you've done something, yet you've probably not taken in

too many calories. This method of eating (a little at a time, rather than three huge meals a day) is highly desirable simply because it is so NATURAL.

If you want to really make a meal of nuts, you might want to try them with bits of dried fruits. You may know this concoction by the popular name of GORP. Some of us at the Center For Human Natural Nutrition have spent many days in the forest or desert eating NOTHING but Gorp and feeling quite satisfied nutritionally, under rigorous conditions.

2. Another method is to try chopping or even mashing them as a filler, with Hunza Bread, eating them in a crunchy kind of sandwich. You'll be surprised at how tasty this will be. Nuts are also a good additive in that 'super salad' mixture for a special occasion.

3. By using a food processing machine, you can change the entire texture of the nut (peanuts and almonds are standard favorites) and make ' nut-butter'. Obviously, with bread , honey and a little juice you'll have a complete meal that will satisfy your every need.

YOUR FOOD AND FIRE

We have been conditioned to cook every food item. Not only do we cook our vegetables, green leaves, beans and legumes, we even cook our fruits and roast & toast our nuts and seeds.

To cook any human natural food, in reality, means changing the properly balanced nutrition that was contained in it with heat, one of natural physics most powerful reactions. Heat is one fundamental way that Nature has of changing things. With the process of applying heat the Creator allows us to turn ice to water and water to steam, for instance. It is one universal way of 'disinfecting' as well. This simply means that not much can survive prolonged, high temperatures. This is true of the live, nutritional elements in your foods, too.

When we cook our foods, the enzymes that are present (and make our food LIVE to begin with) are killed and destroyed. The living part of the foods we eat are the most vital for the human body, and unfortunately some of the most fragile.

Enzymes, for instance will be destroyed at temperatures of 130 degrees and above. This is not as hot as you might think. The surface of our streets in cities like Los Angeles, regularly exceed this temperature every summer. Desert air temperature of many lands throughout the world, often reach this temperature. Even the lowest setting on your oven can easily sustain a temperature of 130 degrees.

It is important to remember, due to the fragility of enzymes, that any food you cook at temperatures in excess of 130 will not be as health producing as those eaten raw or cooked at lower temperatures. Raw, fresh, live food will always be your best choice, but we realize that (as humans) our conditioning to cook foods (established since the Ice Age) is very strong. You will probably have a strong craving for cooked foods, even if you 'know' that you shouldn't eat them, and even if you LIKE the tastes of Raw foods.

Using our 'informal poll' around the Center, we've discovered an interesting phenomenon. Most of us prefer Raw Foods when we are in natural settings. In other words, when we have the chance to camp out or be in nature for a day or two, raw, natural, live foods are our preference. But, when we are in a modern, City setting, our cravings become modern. It's almost as if our inner voice, when placed in an atmosphere 'close to the way the Creator intended for us' speaks louder and more clearly than when drowned out by the sounds of automobiles and heavy machinery. This is only natural, and one of the reasons why we suggest going to the mountains, or desert or sea shore as much as possible.

In regard to cooking though, don't allow this to be the source of new stresses. We have been CONDITIONED to like cooked foods and we CAN be reconditioned.

So, here are some general ideas on how to prepare cooked foods. Later, in our Important Recommendations section we will discuss raw foods as opposed to cooked, and ways to use cooking more moderately.

WHAT YOU SHOULD COOK - AND HOW

The number one thing to remember if you must cook is simply this:The least amount of time at the lowest possible te}perature. Enzymes, like all living things, will have individual tolerance levels. By limiting the time you cook, and/or the temperature you increase the chance that some of the 'hardier' individuals will survive.

To increase the living organisms chances of survival, soak anything that you want to cook in water, overnight (the longer you soak the better) and cook it the next day at the lowest possible setting. The reason for this is that WATER IS LIFE. By adding moisture to the foods you cook, you increase the chances of survival against the drying effects of heat.

In choosing what you'll cook follow these guidelines:

1. Any kind of grains can be cooked and eaten with added oils, spices and sweeteners such as honey, maple syrup or fruit. Technically, when you make Hunza Bread, you are using grain. Another idea for the Dough is to spread it on a large sheet and roll it as thinly as

possible (like a very large pancake). You can add any toppings (more Vegies and Greens, and especially fresh garlic) that you like and what you end up with is a kind of Hunza Pizza!

2. Any kind of beans can be cooked. You can alter the tastes of any bean by adding flavorings (in the form of onion, garlic, spices, oils, juices etc.) WHILE cooking. This has a tendency to put the flavor deeper into the bean, instead on covering it up.

3. Soup is probably the most desirable COOKED food. Vegetable broths are often much more potent suppliers of vitamins and minerals than the vegetable itself (and almost never cause indigestion, even in the most sensitive stomachs). You can make broths from any individual or combination of vegetables and ingredients. And, remember, when you are cooking vegetables DON'T THROW OUT THE WATER! Drink it down. It, in fact, is just the broth that you'd make soup from and has all the vitamins that you've just cooked away.

When you make soups, blend your desired vegetables in a blender or chop them to your preference. Add natural herbs (go light on the salt) and SIMMER over a low heat. Make sure the cooking pot is covered and don't let the water boil the vegetables for too long (in fact, a steamer is preferable). Add spices if you like and eat the soup UNSTRAINED.

NOTE: Never fry or broil and never use oils when cooking.

These are some very broad and general recipe ideas. For detail and variety, use your imagination, or one of the hundred reference books now available on vegetarian diet. Be cautious, however, most vegetarian diets use dairy products, eggs or chemicals. Theses are not what you want.

THE DAILY AND WEEKLY DIET PROGRAM

1. DAILY SCHEDULE : Every day, on a regular basis, you must comply with the following schedule. This is a "must" program.
a) The first thing in the morning you must take your "Morning Freshener." This includes: One glass of fresh fruit juice (orange, grapefruit) mixed with one fresh lemon juice.
b) Three medium carrots to be grated (net weight of eight to ten ounces) with one or two teaspoons of honey, mixed and eaten.
 c) Three times daily (any time during the day, with meals preferred) you must take, each time one big or two medium clove of fresh garlic or the equivalent in garlic capsules.
d) During the day (preferably in the morning and early afternoon) take 500mg. to 1500mg.of Bee Pollen.

2. Last thing before sleeping, your "Nightly Cleansing" is part of this "must" program and it includes: One fresh lemon juice to be mixed with one or two cups of warm/hot water or herb tea and one or two teaspoons of honey.

3. Weekly eating schedule :   We have five food groups that must be eaten on a regular basis: vegetables, green leaves, fruits, grains & beans and nuts & seeds. If you eat three (small and large) meals of breakfast, lunch, and dinner a day, then for the total in a week you will have 21 meals.
a) You must schedule your meals in a manner that you will eat, as evenly as possible, from the five food

groupings. Let us say, for the whole week you eat almost four from each group.

b) A weekly eating schedule might look like the chart below, but you can arrange your own schedule to suit your own taste and convenience. If you want to leave out any one meal, then, by all means, do it. In fact, this short break in eating is a small 'fast' that is quite healthful and cleansing.

c) Some people like the idea of eating before going to bed, though, because it gives them the feeling that they're full. These same people complain that dieting always fails because they can't think about anything but food. We don't want you to lose sleep over your meals. On the other hand, if you can avoid eating before going to bed it's great. If you can't, then by all means, what you'll be eating is far better for you than what you're probably used to.

d) Because you will be taking your Morning Freshener, therefore for breakfast we have scheduled Nuts or Fruits. If you wish, you can combine the Morning Freshener and your breakfast.

	Breakfast	Lunch	Dinner
Monday	F	G	V
Tuesday	N	GL	F
Wednesday	F	G	GL
Thursday	N	V	F
Friday	N	GL	V
Saturday	F	V	G
Sunday	N	G	GL

V=Vegetables   GL=Green leaves   F=Fruits
G=Grains & Beans   N=Nuts & Seeds

4. If you can not follow our recommended schedule then arrange your own eating schedule according to the principles we've set down in previous sections of this

book. Use any of the five groupings, but remember,that the more variety and greater number of food groups that you eat daily, the better results you can expect. This is logical since each group tends to serve certain needs. And, while it is true that one Super Healthy Meal a week is better than five empty, toxic conventional meals; the more consistent you are in your supply of nutrients, the better able your body will be to correct mistakes and heal itself on the regular basis that it needs.

So, as for variety, when making fruit salad, use as many kinds of fruits as possible. Apply this same principle to your vegetable salads, leaf portions and the others.

5. For each meal, it is advisable not to mix different food categories. Try to eat from only one food category at a time. This means if you eat fruit do not eat grains or beans in the same eating session. Allow two or three hours of time between eating from the various food groups. This will allow your body time to adjust any new ingredients in your diet (some might not agree with you, or cause reactions because you're not used to them--we will discuss this phenomenon at a later time).

6. To produce the very best results you will want to nourish your body on live, fresh, raw, ORGANICALLY GROWN vegetables, green leaves, fruits, nuts, grains and beans. Regardless of your present health status, if you adhere to these principles and follow the TEN COMMANDMENTS OF HEALTH, you should be rewarded with a gift that the Creator intended for all people...supreme health, marked by endless energy, resulting in a long, happy life.

7. Try to reduce your cooked food intake. If you cannot resist the craving for hot, cooked food, try to satisfy these annoying cravings with as little as you can.

However, keep in mind, if you want to make progress, you cannot take one step forward and two backward, as the saying goes. To feel a difference,we recommend that you keep the ratio of your raw food intake to well over 80% of your total diet. Also, using the same analogy, you can't expect improvements in your progress if you take GIANT steps backward, more often than you take forward ones. This means that it would not do you much good to try raw foods for one day, then binge on chocolate cakes, coffee and fatty beef another six.

The higher the raw food percentage OF YOUR TOTAL food intake, the better the result. And, this is going to take some time--this will vary according to your present, personal condition, as well. We are assuming (with the enclosed dietary recommendations) that all of your 21 weekly meals are of equal volume. With this in mind, approximately two meals during the week will comprise a little over 10% your total weekly diet. Some quick figuring shows us that these two meals are your SAFETY MARGIN. They are the amount that you can allow yourself for error and still expect positive results (assuming also that you are not starting off with other serious handicaps).

8. When organizing your menu, make sure that the specific items listed in the following chart are used....and used GENEROUSLY. Make certain, too that these items appear in your diet on a REGULAR basis. In the transition period of cleansing and healing that your body will be going through for a time, it is especially important that you use these items regularly as there is an abundance of vital nutritional elements contained in each that will greatly aid in your bodily system's fight to cleanse itself. These items are, therefore considered to be

VERY POWERFUL CLEANSING and HEALING AGENTS:

VEGETABLES	GREEN LEAVES	FRUITS
Carrots	Spinach	Lemon
Cabbage	Kale	Orange
Garlic	Radish leaves	Grapefruit

GRAINS	NUTS	MISC.
Sprouts of all kinds	Peanuts	Honey
Oat bran	Almond	Olive oil
Rice Bran	Pine Nuts	Bee Pollen

9. If you have a serious illness or a degenerative disease and intend to stop it or heal yourself by changing your diet, ask the opinion of those who have taken similar action. They will all tell you that in such situations you MUST MAINTAIN A 100% strict diet of RAW LIVE FOODS.

Among all the wonderful, life giving foods that are contained here, Lemon Juice, Carrots, Garlic, Rice Bran, Oat Bran, Raw Spinach, Kale and Sprouts are highly important for cleansing and healing. If you are interested in quickly changing your current health standard to one of more vibrant and energetic health, then eat these regularly and in generous portions. Also make it a habit to nibble a good amount or drink a lot of juices so that you get input from the other categories.

Before leaving this section, we wanted to make one last comment about a food that has gotten a good deal of media attention lately. This food is Oat Bran. If you are already using Oat Bran on a regular basis, good. It is one time when commercial business interests were set to work in a healthful direction. Because someone got the idea to sell Oat Bran (which was at one time, interestingly, considered to be barely fit for cattle) to the general public, many people have added an important source of fiber (low in sodium and high in complex carbohydrates) to their diets. Three cheers for progress. At least in this one case, we actually have movement in a positive direction. Let's be happy for every step forward though. Those of us who've been working to educate on matters of health and ecology can use all the encouragement we can get.

SUMMARY

This book, thus far, has tried to emphasize that we CAN take control of our health and make changes for the better. As a powerful example of our premise, we've presented a very important, PROVEN, and we believe, desirable lifestyle of a community of people as a model for a viable alternative to our own mixed up way of living. The alternative that we've presented is not a 'vague idea', but a workable pattern that has been tested over many generation the ten COMMANDMENTS of HUNZA health are all important aspects of the overall health picture of the Hunzakuts. Some, however, are more important than others. Eating the right kinds of foods--treating the subject of nourishing your body with respect--is one of the more important messages that we are trying to convey.

The relative recommendations that we've made, in regard to food do not represent suggestions of a 'temporary' nature. All dietary recommendations are permanent ones, part of an overall blueprint for a new lifestyle.

The basic principles of our food recommendations are to use a wide variety of items from the five food groups, on a regular daily basis. ABANDON ALL UNNATURAL FOODS, including toxic, chemicalized, processed and other conventional foods. This is the only way you'll know that your body is GETTING and is able to USE the full nutritional value of the food (fuel) consumed. You'll rest assured, in other words, that you are giving your body all that it requires for vibrant health.

In the meantime, by abstaining from conventional foods, you'll also know that you're not continuing to supply your body with unnecessary and harmful toxic materials (more than we are already subjecting it to as dominant forces in our modern, advanced life-style).

You should worry, for now ONLY about eating right, following the path that was set down for us by the Creator. If we trust the 'system' then we can leave all the rest to the Natural Healing Powers of live, natural foods and the Natural Doctor within our own bodies to assure that disease and misery will be things of the past in our lives.

Finally, if you think that the recommendations that we've given for your diet are too radical to continue on a life-long basis, please do not despair. Simply try the diet, adhere to the recommendations for a TRIAL PERIOD and evaluate for yourself the effectiveness of what we've said. Let your inner voice, in the form of Common Sense, guide you in your decisions. The healthy experience that you will see might convince you that you can no longer tolerate a harmful and unhealthful diet and lifestyle, and you will look for even more information on how to STAY HEALTHY. We are supplying you with all the needed information to maintain a healthier and happier life. You may choose to become healthier, healthiest or achieve the ultimate health.

This book, along with accompanying literature will give you options of different levels of health that you can maintain. It will also give you alternatives for varying degrees of health, with suggestions on efforts to achieve these health standards. For instance, to be healthier than the average person in our society is very easy. It will recommend simply to avoid a few conventional foods. The extreme alternative would be to adhere to a strict diet of highly nutritional, natural foods which will result in a life free of disease and blessed with extreme vitality, endless energy, and completely outside the realm of our present, conventional health standards. It is your body, your health and ultimately YOUR CHOICE. Obviously, you are the best person to decide not only which standard of health you want to strive for, but what you think you can achieve. In any case, you must KNOW YOURSELF, and honestly consider the effort you are willing to make to achieve your goals.

This is why there are TEN COMMANDMENTS for ultimate health. Following just one Commandment is not enough, but It's a start.

CHAPTER SEVEN

FACTS AND TESTIMONIALS

Ever since the people of Hunza were 'discovered' by scientists of the western world these simple, gentle people have been subjected to every manner of probe, study and indignity. Instead of looking at them as a 'community' with a workable model of behavior for the improvement of health for all humanity, they have been treated either as guinea pigs or suspects in a gigantic hoax. Those who come looking to uncover the lie, are the biggest fools of all. They sit in the middle of an incredible atmosphere, with beauty all around them, and concentrate on finding only ugliness. These people (who've never found any real evidence of wrongdoing other than one woman who was mistaken about her birthday...over 100 years ago) deserve no more than this brief mention and our pity.

On the other hand, the scientific searchers are not much better. Many have come with good intentions, but are just as blind as the amateur 'detectives'. Inevitably they go away from their experience in Hunza with a new found sense of respect, but varying answers as to the source of the Hunzakuts incredible energy, extraordinary health and longevity. But, as usual, science has been looking for too complicated an answer to very simple questions. This is like not being able to see the forest, because you've decided to try and 'discover' a single tree.

For the most part, research has centered around trying to locate the 'one special substance' in the soil, air, water or food that is unique to the area and will account for the incredible health of these people.

It's sad that medical science hasn't looked for the simple answer first. Often, in fact, the simple solution is never even considered, because, if they were found, then there would be really no need for the profession of "BIG MONEY" scientific investigation at all.

In Hunza, there has been no need of doctors (or witch doctors) for countless generations. What need is there for such a thing when no one gets sick?

But, instead of examining this fact in an honest and fair light, the medical and 'scientific' trade has, over thousands of years, been conditioning the public to ignore their own belief and wisdom (the Inner Voice) and to put their entire faith (and lives) in the hands of technology. This one group (those concerned with medicines and magical answers) has given rise to an ever mushrooming medical profession. A group that now, not only has taken control of our lives, but would like us to believe that THEY know better than the voice of the spirit that the Creator has given to us all. And, in this confused and distorted wandering there is the added problem that we now have of various sub-sciences' or disciplines. It used to be that the search for truth was simply, the search for truth. Today, the search has been broken up into hundreds of little searches, with each person and group guarding every bit of knowledge they might gain, from every other individual and group. The Anthropologists don't want the Sociologists to get to 'who knows where?' first. And, the physicists NEVER tell the Chemists what they've learned. Good heavens! The Chemists might use that knowledge to come up with something USEFUL. Maybe, even the TRUTH will be discovered. Then what? Chaos would reign. Wouldn't it?

If you wonder why they guard every bit of information they uncover from others, again we come back to commercialization. They wish to keep the economic advantage of that information or finding to themselves or their group. Only in that way can they hope to reap ALL the economic benefits for themselves.

So, scientists,in an effort to promote their own sense of self importance, continue to search for the magical element, from their own narrow perspectives, to determine what the elixir is that's responsible for the health of the people of Hunza. And, due to this atmosphere of back-biting and in-fighting and closely guarded secrets, each individual group continues to ignore that the amazing longevity and vitality of these people is merely the result of a more natural lifestyle, one in accordance with the laws of the Creator. The people of Hunza nourish themselves with a very high percentage of raw, fresh and live foods, seclude themselves from the stresses of technology and are mostly protected (due to circumstance and location) from the chemicals that tend to dominate our Modern Life.

THE DOMINATION OF CHEMICALS

To emphasize how strongly we feel about the domination of chemicals over our lives, we need only look at what has already been said concerning the quality of air, water and food in most major cities of the world. Daily warnings are posted in newspapers and presented on T.V. and radio about the dangers of such hazards as Breathing, Drinking and Eating.

This endless barrage is a 'two edged sword' for the promoters of healthy products and lifestyles. On the one hand people are definitely more health conscious now than for any period in the past 2000 years. But, most of them see the situation as so hopeless that they give up in despair and don't try to change things. We need a sense of urgency AND courage; so, we can take action to improve the total situation. In that way alone, can we benefit.

Needless to say, other than chemicals, which are present in every food item we consume (to varying degrees), we consider coffee, soft drinks, alcohol, tobacco, sugar, white flour, animal fat and processed foods to be equally hazardous to human health. The validity of this statement has been verified more than once, even by the many 'disciplines' of modern science. These substances are now known by ALL to be major causes of cardiovascular disease, cancer and many other problems. Again, the United States' own Surgeon General C. Everett Koop, has taken the role of Head Health Honcho to heart, crusading (almost rabidly at times) for the return to common sense, and the elimination of animal fats, chemicals and other unnatural substances from our diets and lifestyle. This matter is of monumental importance, and the Surgeon General has shown some courage to speak out. His courage is especially apparent since (being a Government Official) he is certainly pressured by special interest groups not to say anything negative about their products.

Some of us, in an attempt to combat the chemical onslaught on our bodies, spend hours searching the supermarket shelves for those 100% natural packages. This also has, unfortunately become a source of despair for many of us. For, when we locate those searched for packages, we discover that this is just another case of false advertising. We should NOT despair however. Even though we know that we're being lied to in many cases, we also know that health is returning to the forefront of the attention of Big Business. If we can keep the moneygrubbers on the track of health, eventually we might even convince them that TRULY 100% NATURAL is what will make them the most money. When that time comes, we'll all profit.

Until that time comes, however, be skeptical. You might even think that fresh produce in a supermarket is exempt from toxification. This, however, is not true either. The produce that many of us consider to be fresh is really inundated with chemicals from the time the seed is packaged until harvest. Our produce is so heavily contaminated from soil additives, chemical fertilizers, sprays, powders and pesticides that it is a wonder anything will grow at all.

To understand just how damaging these chemicals are to our living foods, we can try a simple test for ourselves. The next time you are in one of those 'under-developed countries' where chemicals are not used so extensively (because they can't afford them--and must actually work to produce foods) or if you have the opportunity to try some TRULY organically grown vegetables and fruits, you'll certainly see a vast difference in aroma and taste from what you've been getting in the supermarkets. One of the Center's volunteers tells a story about a friend who had a bunch of citrus trees in his backyard (planted years before his friend had moved in). But, the friend didn't even think to use the fruit that was produced there. One particularly hot day in summer, they were talking about making some 'fresh lemonade' and the friend said he'd have to go the store and buy some lemons. "But, you have lemons right here!" Our volunteer pointed out. It never crossed this guys mind that the fruit that grew in his yard was edible, let alone BETTER than the fruit he could spend money on. The volunteer said that he even had a 'heck of a time' convincing his friend that the lemons were O.K. to eat if they came off a tree and not off a shelf. "I had to eat one of them to prove that they weren't poison."

The conditioning to pollute ourselves at the expense of our Common Sense, is everywhere and very powerful. In addition to our air pollution, chemicalization of water and contamination of foods, consider the toxic wastes that we subject our bodies to in the form of pain killers and drugs, mouthwash and soaps, shampoos, conditioners, toothpastes, antiperspirants, and perfumes. Many of us even fill the air of our immediate surroundings with even more pollution by using air fresheners, pesticides and other foreign materials that we are not even aware of.

We hope, by this little presentation you will now realize the strength of the phrase 'domination of chemicals'. We'd like you also to realize the responsibility that we possess in regard to other forms of life on this planet. We know, for instance, that our hair spray and other canisters have helped to destroy the Ozone Layer. Also realize that when you make the decision to use polluting detergents in your dishwasher, you are making the choice of destroying the environment a little bit more for the next generation (if there is one). These decisions are based upon pure laziness and a hypnotic hold that advertising has over our lives. You do not have to use polluting shampoos to get your hair 'squeaky clean'. There are plenty of non-polluting shampoos on the market that will do the job every bit as well as the polluters. WE MUST BUY THE BIODEGRADABLE PRODUCTS and make health and ecology PROFITABLE.

One other thing is obtained from an examination of Chemical Domination in our world, and that is an appreciation of the amazing ability of the human body (and all life) to be able to fight off the ill effects of these many unnatural substances. Life is truly a miracle and we should begin treating it as such.

THE SIMPLE LANGUAGE OF COMMON SENSE

Now as we attempt to establish some sound reasons for the exceptional health, longevity and vitality of the people of Hunza, we are going to ask you to do something that may not be comfortable from the standpoint of your recent conditioning. We want you to make your judgments without waiting for the pronouncements from the specialists. We want you to allow your Common Sense to 'check the data' swiftly and accurately. Let's use our Common Sense even at the expense of changing our conditioning.

First, ask yourself the question, "How has this conditioning taken place?"

The process has taken thousands of years and been very effective. For the sake of business, a number of specialized professionals have actually come together to strip the general public of their dollars and their common sense. These professional groups include lawyers, doctors, accountants and so on. Each field has its own special set of regulations, rules, methods and even their own elected Boards who protect the groups interests, forces cooperation & harmony among members and lobbies the legislation for the groups' interests. Within these groups new names, terminologies and even entire languages to make things as complex and intricate as possible are created. In this way, they confuse the general public, preserve their special place in our society and establish their superiority. They STRENGTHEN THEIR OWN MYTH, as it were.

In order to establish this false authority over our lives, it has been necessary to instill in us a desire to avoid taking responsibility for ourselves and our actions. If you have a physical problem, you are told to go to the doctor. If you have a legal problem, you are sent to a lawyer. If your problem is a personal one, you might be directed to a therapist or psychiatrist. In some cases, these special interest groups have worked out a network of expertise. If you have an accident, for instance, you might go to a lawyer, who will send you to a particular doctor and therapist so that your insurance company can collect money from another insurance company.

Experience will tell us that in this game of experts it would not benefit the almighty dollar to send a potential customer away without relieving them of some cash. You will never see one of these experts tell you to 'take care of the problem on your own," unless they think they can't profit in some way. Interestingly, when we do participate in the Game, and seek professional advice, we seldom are assured that our problems will be solved any better than if we'd done our own work and listened to our own Inner Voice. This trend continues however, and because of the interconnections of one business to another business there is a general lessening of the use of Common Sense and an increase in the complications and stresses of modern life.

THE ROLE OF GENETICS

If we summarize the facts presented thus far, our Common Sense will tell us that the reason for the fantastic health of the Hunzakuts stems from their environment and especially their dietary habits. And, this is true. However, our own research has determined that there are other factors involved as well. This is not the 'one special element' that is searched for by other investigators, but it is a factor that contributes to the overall health picture of the Hunzakuts. This answer is genetics. Some have even said that genetics plays the fundamental role in the phenomenon of Hunza Health. Others, even more far out, have gone to the extreme and suggested that the people of Hunza (and all those other healthy communities of the world) are not humans at all, but ancestors of some other race, brought here in spaceships before the time when humans could even stand up straight. This, of course, is just too silly to even grace with a rebuttal and in the end, this kind of nonsense doesn't answer any questions for us--even if it were true.

First of all, there is DEFINITELY something to genetics. We are also willing, to agree that the people of Hunza are genetically superior to the rest of us. But, we think that this question must be further examined. We must remember, these people have been drinking the same healthy water, breathing the same healthy air and eating the same healthy foods for many generations. We know the ancestors of the people of Hunza are Humans, from a not too distant past. So, how is it that they are genetically superior? While living a healthy lifestyle in a healthy environment, a healthy parent will produce healthy offspring (on the whole); Healthy conditions make for the transference of healthy genes; healthy genes make healthy children...and so on. We also have scientific evidence that the contrary is true. A mother can seriously damage the genetic code of her offspring (during development) by using drugs, drinking or smoking...as well as eating improperly.

Remember, however, if we take the Hunzakuts out of Hunza and subject them to all the pollutions and processes that act upon us in an 'advanced society' their health will eventually be diminished. It might take longer for this degeneration to occur to them than someone with 'weaker genes' but it WILL happen. Sooner or later, as we have observed those few individuals who've left Hunza, they will contract all the same diseases that we work so hard to obtain (and in a few cases work twice as hard to avoid) in our modern world.

The ultimate point is that genetics DOES play a role in the overall health of a species AS WELL AS an individual or family. But, we can effectively influence the overall health of a 'gene pool' to the benefit of all, simply by taking care of ourselves, making ourselves healthier,enjoying a world of energy and vitality and passing this energy on (in the form of knowledge AND healthy genes) to our offspring.

PROGRESS WORKS BOTH WAYS

The fact is that the above scenario is exactly what is taking place RIGHT NOW in Hunza. Once these people opened their doors to investigation and progress, an unexpected door was opened to all the ills that we take for granted. Some research, in fact, is specifically geared to the perverted speculation of 'How Long Will The Total Degeneration Of Hunza Take?' Historically speaking, the case of Hunza is exactly the same as dozens of times that modernization destroyed the serenity of a people, culture or environmental system. In the Americas we need to look no further than the landing of Columbus or Cortez to see the exact date when disease and ill health began.

On the environmental front, the destruction of the Rain Forests throughout the world, or the Ozone Layer are daily graphic examples of modernization chipping away (with frightening violence in most cases) at the systems set in motion by the Creator to protect and nurture us.

Thankfully, progress can work both ways. Shortly you will be reading the TRUE LIFE NARRATIVES of the people in our own society (and in our own time) who have taken responsibility for their health and are LIVING PROOF that a return to the use of Common Sense and a harmony with the Laws Of Nature can alter and REVERSE the harmful effects of modernization.

Each individual can only slightly effect the air that they breath and the condition of the water that they drink. These two elements in all of our lives are GLOBAL issues that will take time and continued efforts to change drastically. But, in the meantime every one can drastically change and improve his indoor air and water quality (home & office) where we spend most of our time. We can use a small inexpensive unit to clean and purify the air of the room we most use and with small distillation unit obtain 100% clean and pure water.

Each person who testifies on the following pages and in our other literature, also has other personal limitations that they will specify. But, through partial or intensive adherence to the principles of proper eating, drinking and exercise, they have all achieved amazing results.

Now it is up to you to weigh the facts and consult your Inner Voice or Common Sense for your own benefit as well as the benefit of the whole earth.

Perhaps one day YOU will be one of these amazing individuals who changed the course of their lives through diet and following the other Hunza Health Commandments. If you can make such a change then we are that much closer to the time when WE ALL will be amazingly healthy, and the whole earth will benefit from individual progress.

THE WHOLE TRUTH

A recent 'startling announcement' was made by the National Academy of Science. After an expensive and exhaustive study (no doubt) they determined that a large percentage of disease (40 to 60% was the estimate) could be avoided by simply changing our diets. They suggested limiting fatty meats, whole milk, dairy products and cooking oils in our diets.

Our question is: Why weren't these people able to express the truth COMPLETELY? Why didn't they come right out and say that the food we eat along with the polluted air we breathe, the contaminated water we drink and the lack of physical exercise we get accounts for ALMOST ONE HUNDRED PERCENT of all disease, including cancer, heart attack, arthritis and every other form of illness that is known to mankind?

The reason that they didn't reveal the WHOLE truth becomes obvious when we realize who the first persons were to challenge their findings, even when only a small portion of the truth was revealed. The challengers were people like those in the Meat Industry, the Dairy Industry and the Chemical Industry.

Can you guess what would have happened if the Academy had reported the complete unwatered truth? If they had said that ultimate health comes ONLY when you avoid unhealthy foods, stay away from chemicals and unnatural life-style--that you NEED fresh, raw, live fruits, vegetables, grains and nuts and that packaging and processing and preservatives were unnecessary and harmful?

The uproar would have been tremendous...not from the general public who would've benefited from the truth, but from the Human Health Industry who would've suffered a crippling blow if even 10% of those who currently eat nothing but conventional foods suddenly started eating natural human nutrition. This same industry currently makes hundreds of billions of dollars every year...and, would it surprise you to learn that members of the Academy of Science are actually members and influential constituents of this same Human Health Industry? Perhaps there has been a conflict of interest, you might think. But, NO, there's no conflict. The Academy of Science doesn't care about Human Health or truth. They are only concerned that they will earn their budget projections for the next fiscal year.

And, even if the Academy had been totally honest, there would have been an outcry even louder from another faction. Every large conglomerate industry (The Meat, Dairy, Soda Pop, Coffee, Food Additives, Sugar, Pharmaceuticals and many others) would have been forced to object. That is their right in a free world. And, their objections would probably have come in their usual form, the dreaded lawsuit. Every one of these companies is monstrously large, their profits are enormous and they have but ONE objective. They want even more money than the obscene amounts that they already waste. They have absolutely NO consideration for human life or health. They hypnotize us to purchase their products with mindless advertising then return huge amounts of money back into the task of tricking us further.

With this information in mind, we now present the true life experiences of those individuals who have decided to use their common sense and not base their health decisions merely on recommendations of moneygrubbing experts. Here are some stories, told by those who lived the tales, of how ordinary people such as us, pursue true, natural health and longer, happier lives.

TESTIMONIAL OF KAREN GAIL, WASHINGTON

When I was young, I had the normal, childhood illnesses, such as measles, mumps, colds and flu. We mostly lived on farms during my childhood so I managed to eat enough raw foods. I remember whenever I didn't get enough fresh foods, (mostly during the winter seasons) I generally got sick a lot, or my grades went down in school.

When I was around 12 years old, we moved into Spokane. We ate an over abundance of cooked food, for convenience. A lot of meat, salt, sugar and starchy foods. I gained nearly 20 pounds. I was fat for the first time in my life. I was in a constant state of mental depression, and experienced a lot of illness.

At 15 I had my tonsils and adenoids removed. I had been on starvation diets, off and on, since the age of 13. I was anemic at the time. It took me three months to regain enough strength to stand. Infection had spread through my throat, ears, sinuses and Medulla. (It is still possible to see the damage done in the irises of my eyes.) It took another three months to withdraw from the liquid medicine I had to take every couple of hours. It contained morphine and some other type of drug which caused hallucinations.

When I recovered enough to go back to school, I started taking drugs for any reason I could think of. I managed to find doctors who would write the prescriptions with little or no questions.

I started smoking cigarettes, then marijuana, following the crowd. It later worked into a lot of other drugs.

I got married at 16. We lived in poverty for 2 years (eating bread, potatoes and canned food) before I unexpectedly became pregnant. I was already 25 pounds overweight. I gained about another 25 pounds by the end of the pregnancy.

My labor lasted 48 hours. My son was delivered with the crudest methods. He was born with a lot of allergies, mostly food. He was sick a lot until around age 3, when he outgrew most of them.

I divorced at 19. Trying to make up for lost time, I went on diet pills to lose the last 20 pounds of weight left over from pregnancy. I also took diuretics. I used both [drugs] indiscriminately. On top of that, I began drinking alcoholic beverages quite frequently. I started getting colds and illnesses. Antibiotics became a regular thing. I was using a script about every other week.

One day, I started urinating blood, along with having some serious pain under my ribs on my right side.

My prescriptions for antibiotics was doubled. The pain did not go away though. It just kept getting worse.

I went to different specialists. I had many X-rays taken. Each one said they would probably have to do exploratory surgery to be sure.

One said it was my gall bladder. One said it could be 'liver strings' and they would have to insert a probe through an opening near my navel to see. Another said my liver, kidneys, and bladder were only functioning at about 15 to 20% efficiency. He said things seemed to be deteriorating on the right side of my body only.

I went to see one last doctor. By this time I was thin with no muscle tone, pale with black circles under my eyes. My hair looked like straw. I was having frequent headaches, and was losing more weight because I could not keep any food down.

He asked me some questions and checked me over. His conclusion was a brain tumor. He explained that a tumor can block impulses to the body, making the parts deteriorate after a time. He said that a tumor on the left side of my brain would affect the right side of the body.

I was full of toxic waste, and he said that at the rate my health was deteriorating I probably wouldn't live over another year.

I took the Kelly enzyme test. It was positive. I had a cancerous condition. Surgery was suggested, but I refused. I went home and just accepted my death and felt sorry for myself. Soon, I was so weak I just laid around. Finally, one day out of curiosity, I picked up a book titled, "One Answer To Cancer" by Dr. William Donald Kelley.

It was described how the same digestive aids with chymotripson, used for the test, are used to burn up the cancer. It also explained how cancer could be linked to poor diet and mental attitude. Something signaled inside me. I took it into my own hands from that point on.

I used the digestive aids and began fasting with lemons and herbs. I used different herbs for purifying the blood and to heal certain parts of the body.

I used fresh vegetable and fruit juices. I drank deionized water with liquid trace minerals added.

Fasts lasted 20-40 days at a time, using both herbs and juices. In between the fasts I ate raw vegetables and fruits. The more I fasted, the more my physician within guided me.

I went back to one of the doctors, eight months later. He nearly fainted when he saw me. He noted a vast improvement but did not know whether or not to believe that I did it with nutrition alone. I felt reborn!

Another test showed negative. During and after my illness I studied everything I could get my hands on concerning health and diet. I learned the most through trial and error to get to the diet that I use now. I now eat like people of our ancestry long ago: Leaf, fruit, root and seeds, also sprouts.

This is ideally suited for my body's top performance. Physically, I am more youthful. Mentally, I have raised my I.Q. higher than ever before in my life. Spiritually, I feel like "a natural". And, it keeps getting better everyday!

I occasionally fast now for 10 days at a time. It cleanses the system and heals tired or damaged areas rapidly. At this point, my system is so clean I actually get high from eating the raw foods.

One last thought for anyone afraid to try raw foods. I once read an article about a doctor John Douglas, who delved into ancient scriptures. Chinese, Indian, Hebrew, Greek and Egyptian writings of antiquity all prescribed the same thing:"Cook not" and "Those who cook food, sin as they eat it."

I believe they had a lot less illness and disease back then. Especially for those who loved raw foods.

-Karen Gail

TESTIMONIAL OF NORMAN ZALE, ILLINOIS

About fifteen years ago, after nine years of competitive weight lifting and wrestling, I began to develop arthritis. Every day found me suffering from a new ache or pain:neck, shoulders, elbows, wrists, back, knees and one foot were all involved. I kept on with my weight training and wrestling in spite of the stinging, burning pains. I used no medication, but, in desperation turned to the Natural Hygiene Society. I immediately switched to an all-raw, live food diet (about 90% raw fruits and vegetables, 10% raw seeds, nuts and grains) and to my astonishment, my aches began to vanish within two or three days. After two weeks, all pain disappeared.

I still follow a very similar diet...my strength and endurance is excellent. I still weight lift 4 to 6 days per week, swim one mile three times weekly and perform stretching movements and yoga exercises daily. I also regularly participate in basketball, volleyball, calisthenics and gymnastics. How does one find time for all this physical activity? Well, I have two wonderful jobs, teaching high school physical education (days) and am a Y.M.C.A. program director in the evenings.

-Norman Zale

TESTIMONIAL OF J. NAPIEN SR., MICHIGAN

I was fascinated by the idea of raw foods and after a couple of months of reading everything I could find, I was ready. So, one day the refrigerator was cleaned out of all animal products, totally everything including processed foods. My refrigerator was nearly empty. Though not truly on a raw diet, I felt great the first week then my feelings mellowed for about another week. But, by the third week, I was losing weight and energy fast until one morning I could hardly get out of bed.

I was sick, or so I thought at the time. I went back to 'normal' eating. For about the next seven years I read and followed the health foods fads as they came and went. There were vitamins, herbs, minerals, glandulars, extracts, juice fasts, enemas and a slow conversion to vegetarianism.

During this time, my asthma cleared up. Still the idea of living a more natural lifestyle, and most importantly the idea that humans could live on unfired foods, kept me getting my act slowly together. The big problems was that I was alone in this, or so I thought. It was an August day when I suddenly realized that I was a real raw fooder, for a couple of weeks anyway. Wow, it was so easy, so I just kept going. I lost weight, but I didn't care, I knew what was happening. After a month I became very listless, but I wasn't afraid, I knew I was eliminating toxins. This lasted about two months, coming and going, always though, the highs were getting higher.

Today, I am about 90% or better on raw foods. Whenever I do eat a cooked meal, the next day my eyes, nose and mouth are all mucused.

Hope many more people can be freed from the hocus-pocus of the medical, food and drug cartels. Individuals who can see and realize the benefits of a simple raw food diet, with exercise and good mental hygiene will always be welcomed by mother nature.

--James Napien Sr.

TESTIMONIAL OF KAY VANICA, CALIFORNIA

Three years ago, I learned I had Multiple Sclerosis. Shortly thereafter, I found a nutritionally oriented doctor who suggested I follow a raw food diet. He tested me for allergies and I found that I am allergic to 50% of the natural foods that I ingest. Somewhat discouraged, I was willing to see how raw foods affected my body...They work for me 95% of the time and I sometimes feel weak, and I certainly feel healthier. I feel and know that I am cleansing my body by following the raw food diet.

--Kay Vanica

TESTIMONIAL OF STANLEY C.WEINSIER, FLORIDA

[I was] born in New York City, February, 1910. At 16 years of age, I decided to avoid eating flesh. This was followed by many years of meatless eating while milk and dairy products, and refined breads and cereals were used liberally. Ice cream and sweets were included, because I had no real knowledge of diet. My early years were plagued with hay fever.
By my 21st birthday I had attained a weight of 172 lbs. (plus or minus) and my height of just under six feet handled it pretty well. In the years following, I attempted a few short fasts, the longest being 10 days. In this way I gradually diminished my weight to where I maintained 160 to 165 lbs. for many years. I moved from New York City, to this location in 1936 and started the Health Conservatory here, which has since been changed to the Florida Spa.
Before coming here I had schooled in New York and associated with Dr. Max Warmbrand also of New York.

About the summer of 1958, I had a severe middle ear infection that stopped me in my tracks and made me realize that something was wrong. I then strictly adhered to a severe program of cleansing in an effort to restore the hearing I had lost. From this point on I gave up my brown rice and my baked potatoes and my w.w. bread and cereals and gradually assumed a raw food program.

For many years now, I have been a raw foodist. I eat two meals a day--breakfast about 6 A.M. and dinner about 5 A.M.

Breakfast is a large salad including raw corn and this is followed by whole, raw fruits (no bananas). The evening meal is the same only a little larger. I use approximately 8-9 lbs. of raw food daily and this includes sprouts that I grow. I do not drink fruit juices, I eat only raw fruits in season. This includes citrus, which I grow. But, mostly use apples throughout the winter and spring. Apples frequently number as many as ten in a day.

The question of nuts and seeds I have resolved by using a few nuts very infrequently. This might total a half pound in a year. Sunflower seeds and sesame seeds might exceed this amount slightly. Avocado is used very sparingly, because I believe a very low fat content diet is optimum. My hearing at this time is excellent.

And so, the above gives you an idea of my eating pattern. My health is high and I am active 7 days a week.

--Stanley Weinsier

TESTIMONIAL OF J.R. OGLE, MONTANA

I became a vegetarian in 1970 for reasons which were not entirely medical, so my subsequent increased resistance to disease was an unexpected benefit. My diet has been primarily raw foods for more than ten years now. For the warmer, sunnier half of the year, raw foods comprise 80-85 % of my intake. During colder months I rely more on whole grains so the raw portion of my diet drops to 65-70%.

My susceptibility to chronic bronchitis disappeared shortly after I changed away from the typical American devitalized diet. My weight dropped by twelve pounds, and my complexion and my vision both improved substantially. Most surprising though was the increase in my endurance.

My decision to clean up my daily diet occurred early in my second season of Intercollegiate Track and Field competition. Serious training had already put my weight at what I thought was my ideal racing level. So, a sudden loss of eight percent of my body weight coupled with a relatively sudden gain in distance running ability really astonished me.

Needless to say, I am still running, still a vegetarian, and still enjoying superior health.

--J.R. Ogle

TESTIMONIAL OF LAURA GREEN KINGERY

In high school I began gaining weight. I often had severe stomach pains from worry or over-eating, or both. I always had miserable cramps during my period. I am 5'7" and weighed 145 lbs. But, the worst condition of my ill health as Bulimarexia Nervosa. I was a victim of the psychological eating disorder also called "The Binge Purge Syndrome."

Bulimarexia (as you may know) is the sister sickness to Anorexia Nervosa. Although I never starved myself, (quite the contrary, actually!) I had a serious problem. In my case, I was already paranoid about being rotund, yet had an insatiable appetite. I ate enormous amounts of rich, cooked, often sweet foods. Then, out of guilt and fear of gaining weight, I'd force myself to vomit. Then I would deny myself food for several days and eventually binge again. Not only did the cycle repeat itself,but I began purging everything I ate, knowing most of it was fattening anyway. That's how health food broke my disgusting and shameful habit. I knew I wouldn't get fat or feel stuffed. More on this later. Here's how I discovered my new diet.

I took an interest in exercise classes at the YMCA in my city. I was asked to lead classes, so I really strove to lose weight. I began reading diet and health books. But, no matter what I did, I craved too much food. Fortunately, I met my husband, a pipe designer, who also is a martial artist and vegetarian. I looked into the sort of things he ate, and why, and all I read made a lot of sense. In one day, I decided to stop the abuse I loaded upon my body through my digestive system. I stopped eating meat. I lost ten pounds. My exercising became pleasure. I discovered that the salad I'd eaten before a huge meal could be a meal itself.

Then came my first juice fast. I drank only spring water and juice I made myself for five days. I literally became a new person, and quit eating white flour, sugar, white rice, and all commercially prepared food.

My constant diet, and that of my husband is: Raw fruit, raw vegetables, soup, grains, nuts, seeds, and occasionally raw milk cheeses, yogurt and for him, eggs--fertilized, brown eggs.

I weigh between 120 and 125 pounds. My skin is clear, my eyes are bright blue-green, my hair is thick and shiny, my teeth feel clean. My body feels light, my mind rejuvenated.

Our staple food is salad. These raw produce meals have cured me of obesity, stomach spasms, depression, and most importantly, miserable Bulimarexia Nervosa. I just don't ever feel so full that I want to vomit. And, I don't ever crave junk. (As a matter of fact,the only time I ate some of my mother's cooked something, I felt nauseated.) Most interestingly, I haven't become sick in two years. The only time I saw a doctor, I cured myself. And, you'll be interested in this (I think). I had a yearly pap smear, and the MD said the results showed I had some highly irregular cells within. He started mentioning freezing cells and biopsies. I freaked out. That was just before the time of our biannual fast. (We take two, ten day fasts per year). I took the fast and returned for a re-exam two weeks later. Whatever had caused the cell irregularity had vanished. The doctor was pleased, but when I tried to tell him what I believed the fast had done, he became belligerent, sarcastic and blunt. I have not been to a doctor since.

Raw foods/health foods have cured several other illness that I had earlier understood to be 'part of life'. Before my first fast, I took allergy shots twice a week for allergies to trees, grasses, mold and mildew, animal dandruff, dust and tobacco. I quit taking the shots for the fast, and have not missed them, period! Associated with the allergies were sore throats I had at least twice a year. I always needed some sort of shot for them. No more sore throat, or itchy nose, or watery eyes! And I still have menstrual cramps, but they are slight in comparison to what they had been. My cure now is plenty of calcium, blackstrap molasses, B-6 and raw papaya. (Papaya will cure practically any stomach ailment as well).

I'd also like to say that becoming a raw vegger has cleared my mind in some way. I have a greater understanding of life; less worry about daily problems. I have a great desire for pure food, and appreciate the taste of raw produce. I feel energetic, intelligent, happy. I am able to grasp "Way Out" concepts, adapting many as normal behavior for my husband and me. As far as I and my husband are concerned...there is just no alternative to diet. There is no turning back.

--Laura Green Kingery

TESTIMONIAL OF RAY E. NASSER, CALIFORNIA.

In 1970, after being back from Viet Nam for over a year, I began to experience some unusual health problems which did not seem to be resolved by traditional western medicine, as practiced at the V.A. hospitals I went to for health. My digestive system was chronically upset; I was very susceptible to colds and felt generally run down, tired and depressed. I finally received help from a friend who had been to a naturopathic doctor. My friend suggested that I try a raw food diet...The first two weeks were the hardest.
I started win an apple-juice and herbal tea fast then ate nothing but vegetables, raw fish, nuts, grains and fruits. My body seemed to rebel to the new regimen and strange new foods. But, after one month I was feeling very energetic. I also began to enjoy my food and the whole dining process...I have been eating this way for over eleven years now, and will never go back to my old habits of large quantities of fried meats, processed foods, sugar, etc. I am healthy and feel I am growing healthier and stronger each day. I suggest that anyone who has chronic health problems investigate a whole food and/or raw food diet. It may be rough at first, but given a chance, the person may find this is really the only way to eat and live well.

Ray E. Nasser

CHAPTER EIGHT

THE RELATIONSHIP OF SCIENCE AND DISEASE

It is generally believed that there is a direct, positive relationship between scientific advances (especially those in medicine) and the number and frequency of diseases. In other words, the general public thinks that as science advances, more people will live longer AND be more healthy, and that there will be less pain, disease and agony overall. There is even the projected belief that someday, if science and medicine are allowed to reach their pinnacles all suffering will be swept from the face of the earth forever. Through science, it is thought, we can 'return to the Garden Of Eden' on Earth.

This concept is flawed to the point that it is a complete deception. If we examine the statistical information that is available, and use our Common Sense, we will see that exactly the opposite is true. In other words, the more we rely on technology and science, the FARTHER from Eden (natural perfection) we will get.

Over the last few decades, more and newer diseases (ones that we never thought possible a hundred years ago) have begun to deliver effective blows to the human race. This is especially apparent in the more advanced societies such as the United States. Much of the damage done has now trickled out of our own race and is detrimentally effecting the entire world.

What is interesting is that, within this shadow of destruction that we've surrounded ourselves with, humans have become convinced that the propaganda about science making all things wonderful is correct. We have, as a species and especially in countries like the U.S. developed a kind of 'health arrogance'.

Certainly, we've never been shy about showing our pride in being human. We brag about 'how intelligent' we are, how industrious etc. All creatures are measured in relationship to 'how much like us' they are. The problem that exists today is that this arrogance has grown to include every aspect of our existence. At first we believed that the Creator put all knowledge and skill at our disposal. Now, we have convinced ourselves that we've actually put these superior mental and physical abilities to work achieving the very highest levels of every phase of life.

This physical arrogance is especially interesting coming from a creature that cannot run even as fast as a Hippopotamus, does not swim well (nor does the skill come naturally), has less endurance than most every other creature on earth, has relatively poor eyesight, extremely limited hearing and the weakest muscles of all the apes (a chimpanzee is smaller, but about ten times stronger). What do we really have going for us? An ability to use our thumbs and to reason. The first ability we've given over to tasks such as tennis and the second we've relinquished in favor of comfort.

So, now, our biggest brags are reserved for the most typically human pursuits of all...science and technological advancement.

HEALTH AND THE 'LOWER SPECIES'

In light of all the bragging that goes on, let's examine the   health of the animal world in relationship to humanity. If we can find a few places on earth where the bungling interventions of mankind (a sign, no doubt of superiority) has yet to destroy the environment completely, we can see just how well the animals take care of themselves.

Man, and rightly so, has long believed himself to be superior to the other creatures on the planet.   The problem is that we have lost sight of who granted this superiority, and what form it was supposed to take. Our original purpose on Earth (according to the many scriptures) was to act as caretakers of the earth and its inhabitants. Unfortunately, we lost sight of our original harmonious involvement with the Creator's plan very early on in our existence. We have now confused our superior reasoning ability and our added responsibility to watch over the Creator's plan, with a 'separateness' from the plan which evolved us.   We've now taken our superiority and worked feverishly to expand and complicate our achievements by using science and technology as a replacement for our interaction with the inner voice.

In the wild areas of the world, we will find deer, lions, elephants and other creatures who are not 'taken care of' by man. These animals live their lives totally governed by the laws of nature. In these rare cases, we will notice that there are no wild animals suffering from heart disease, cancer, kidney failure, high blood pressure or the most common ailments of humanity, the common cold and flu.

It is a subtle irony that those animals that we pay the most attention to (the ones who we say are benefiting from science and technology) are precisely the ones who suffer the most. The domesticated animal is the one that gets all the ailments that humans have come to accept such as colds, flu, arthritis, heart disease, etc. Of course, humans have found another way to make a buck and since we do see animals getting sick, we now have an wholly modern phenomenon in the invention of animal doctors (the veterinarian). Veterinarians have become one of the strongest political voices and best paid professions in the nation, in fact. What we've failed to realize though is these animals would not contract disease if they hadn't been contaminated, in some way by people.

Additionally, the so called 'wild creatures' who have the most problems are those whose lives have become entangled with Civilization. Animals in the wild must now add to their list of concerns 'protecting themselves from humanity.' The WAY that we jeopardize the lives of our natural creatures can come in many forms. Our mismanagement could take the form of an oil spill, for instance, or a chemical dump in our waterways that kills hundreds of thousands of animals in the matter of just a few days. Or, our 'mistakes' could be ones, such as chemical spraying on vegetables, or poison gases which destroy many species over longer periods of time and are then put into our atmosphere to affect ALL LIFE from then on. The numbers of California Condors (which are suffering now due to high concentrations of Lead in the animals that it eats) is down to a critical 40 birds (all in Zoos at this time). This creature performs a function that nature needs and wants. It cleans up our messes. But, even our mess has become so toxic that the Condor has been poisoned out of performing its vital role in the Plan.

The fact is that Natural Selection takes care of its species by ridding itself of disease. When an individual animal gets a disease in nature, or has somehow gotten itself out of the flow of health with the others of its species, it usually dies, ending the possibility of infecting others.

If a species' existence becomes detrimental to OTHER life forms, threatening to effect them in a negative way, nature usually steps in to destroy that species completely. Extinction, prevents a species from conflicting with the others that are living in harmony. The dinosaurs didn't make it for some reason, and some believe that HUMANS are polluting themselves out of existence altogether too. In our obsession to 'populate the earth' we've all but covered the entire surface with signs of our 'superiority'. The result is that our existence has so interfered with the natural processes, that animals never have a chance to become extinct according to their unfitness with the natural harmony. In other words, the 'Natural Laws never have a chance to decide what species is 'doing its job' and which are not, because WE are making them ALL extinct first. Recent estimates, alarmingly are as high as 10,000 species A DAY, destroyed by man's wanton destruction of the environment. Some individuals appease themselves with the argument that,"these figures are exaggerated by the environmentalists" (a word that should be thought of as very good, but the money grubbers have perverted it to be synonymous with evil).

First of all, those who call themselves environmentalists can exaggerate. But, we feel that it doesn't matter. At least the Environmentalists are taking sides with the earth and the natural processes. Secondly, it doesn't matter if these estimates are exaggerated by ten times. We don't have the right to destroy even ONE OTHER SPECIES OF LIFE, especially since the Creator gave US life to protect these other creatures!

So, human disease is a reward of human life. Certain ailments are reserved for those animals that mankind has 'saved' from an involvement with mother nature in order that these animals can be 'company' for man, or so that they can provide some sort of other commodity to fuel the continuing struggle of building a superior race. In either case, the perversion of the Creator's original plan is obvious.

THE INFECTION OF MAN'S ARROGANCE

First, man separated himself from nature, then he strived to cover up his evil deed in his own mind, finally he took it upon himself to systematically separate all other species of life on the planet from their natural habitat and the natural laws.

Additionally, we compound our own problems in the area of health, the more that we meddle in the natural process of life with our own domesticated animals. We feed our cattle, chickens, dogs and cats commercially processed foods and chemicals, or we allow them to feed on foods that we've poisoned with our unnatural cultivation practices.

In both cases, as technology progresses and business interests gain a stronger hold in our lives, different formulas have been prepared for our animal helpers. As a result, a conglomerate of chemicals (either through fertilization, injection, or direct feeding) has served to replace, entirely, the natural foods of our animals as well. Thus, varying diseases have a stronger hold on our humanly infected, domesticated animals.

The point here is twofold. Even if meat were edible (which it isn't), it certainly couldn't be nutritious now that we've turned our livestock into steroid filled balloons of chemicals. The hunting of healthy, wild, live animals in a spiritual manner (as our American Ancestors did), showing respect for the killed beast to the point of thanking it for allowing you to kill it, is FAR different from hitting caged animals over the head with hammers after depriving it of any resemblance of natural life.

There is another category of animal that also contracts disease, thanks to its unfortunate involvement with humans. These are the laboratory animals, the sorrowful mice, rabbits, monkeys, dogs and the like who are raised (sometimes from birth) in a totally unnatural environment merely for vain, human experimental purposes. These sad creatures are pumped full of chemicals (sugar, fats, saccharine, white flour and others too horrible to imagine) simply to see what will happen. This is extremely perverse, as we already know in almost every case the result of the tests. It's no wonder that these animals end up with all the diseases of modern humankind including (but not limited to) kidney disease, heart failure, cancer and diabetes. If we ate the ratio of chemicals-to-body-weight that we inject some of these creatures with, we'd die even more quickly than we do. It's unbelievable that some of these investigations continue to be financed by our tax dollars. If we'd just ask our Common Sense for verification, it would be happy to tell us that chemicals cause cancer. We don't need to torture animals to verify this. And, the sad part of this whole construction is that these animals are being tested (tortured) in the name of improving HUMAN health and lives. This is one of the greatest deceptions of the century.

The fact is that these scientist and the sponsoring companies and government agencies are merely trying to find new ways to make money. In a market that thrives on using more and more chemicals, the researcher's job is to pump an animal full of chemicals or offending foods, make the animal sick (which is no surprise) and then find NEW chemical formulas that will cure the disease or symptoms that the CHEMICALS caused in the first place.

Let's make no mistake, we are not arguing the mental superiority of the human race. Every species has something special about itself and our reasoning processes are our specialty. We are merely asking, "What have we got to show for our bragging?"

It is not enough to have this mental superiority. We have to learn to use our special God-Given Talent, in a way that was intended by the Creator. If we look where our arrogance is leading us, can we truly brag about our accomplishments? Certainly, science and medicine keep coming up with newer gadgets and ways of doing things. Often, these great new inventions, really do help individuals. One example of this help would be the invention of a mechanical hand or foot for an accident or amputee victim. Science is tremendous at fixing broken parts of bodies, such as replacing hips or bones.

But, if you think about it, there are so few who really benefit from these advancements, mainly due to the fact that "somebody's got to pay for all this". If you don't have insurance or lots of extra money, then the mechanical hand will always be just a dream for you. In addition, many of the so called breakthroughs in 'body repair' are necessary BECAUSE of science. We wouldn't have to now **repair** a faulty heart valve if we didn't **mess up** the heart with 'science' and other unnatural contributions to begin with. But, we'll elaborate on that in a moment.

THE ENDLESS ROAD OF RESEARCH

The thing that is particularly disturbing is that all of this 'research' and all the animal suffering that goes on in its name, takes place merely to buy time (and more profits) for the additive and chemical businesses.

In fact, food additives (known to be a significant factor in the creation of human disease) are estimated to now make up about 80% of our total diet. While this chapter was being written, a television news report said that there are now over 2,000 food additives on the market, but of these that are in common use, only 4 out of every 100 have ever been tested!

Aside from the fact that the results of these few tests are being continually challenged by the industries involved, each day 25 more additives are being created (and used) than the number that get proper testing. Before science ever completes even one cycle of tests we may well be eating NOTHING but chemicals.

And why do we let this happen? Mostly our destruction is due to laziness, according to one report in the April 16th edition (1989) of the Daily News. A scientist (actually, one of those crazy environmentalists), Jill Ratner in an article entitled, Assault On Earth, points out that most of our woes are the result of our being lazy. "Most people," says Ratner, "tend to point the finger of blame on the other guy. When, in truth {our} problems begin with a lifestyle intent solely on convenience."

And, while we suffer with new diseases and destructions of our environment the debates, retesting and counter-results continue to lead us nowhere and prove nothing.

ANOTHER CASE IN POINT

To further illustrate where humanity is leading itself with its arrogance and bragging about scientific advancement, let's see what's taken place with a food item that is so basic to mankind that it is closely associated with civilization.

A recent alarm was sent out by farming communities throughout the world, that the WHEAT plant, through centuries of hybridization and unnatural domestication, has lost almost all of its natural ability to fend off disease. We finally got our wish, a plant that can literally not exist without us. But is that so great?

Some of those who still consult their Common Sense seem to think not, and are trying to figure out what to do about the problem. One suggestion for attempting to revitalize this highly cultivated grain was to reintroduce it to other wild grains, allowing it to cross pollinate with them. In other words, it became obvious that a way was needed to help this plant (that we've succeeded in cutting off from nature altogether) 'return to nature' as a method of regaining its inbred immunizations to disease.

What science and technology has done to wheat (both before and after the harvest) is symbolic of how they think and treat the human body. We know that wheat is now almost completely unable to protect itself from disease and relies completely on humans for every aspect of its existence.

We treat the human body the same way we treat our commercially grown wheat. It is no surprise that we get A.I.D.S. (total break down of our immune system) while our wheat, becomes totally unable to defend itself against disease. Isn't it interesting while at the same time very alarming? It is interesting because it demonstrates that THE LAWS OF NATURE works for humans the same way they work for all other live things. If you live outside these LAWS (which are designed by a higher power) you will pay for it. If you force innocent wheat to follow in your footsteps, then the wheat has to pay for it, by becoming defenseless against any disease. Is it not the time for us to brag a little more about our achievements? We have just created a situation where our wheat has to join the "modern society" of contracting A.I.D.S.

But, getting back to the wheat, after it is harvested, the meddling of human hands continues. First, the wheat grain is stripped of its most important nutritional element by the removal of the bran (actually, if you are willing to pay extra you can now find wheat products with the bran left in). The germ of the wheat (the living part of the seed) is destroyed or discarded. What is left? The wheat center, which is mostly starch with very few distinctive vitamins. This lifeless form is then further processed into flour; chemicals are added, and this is presented to the public as white, high quality, enriched flour.

How can a food be enriched when all the original, wholesome, natural, living nutrition is taken out of it and chemicals are substituted for the enzymes, vitamins, minerals and proteins? There is an old saying that you can't go in two directions at the same time. The logic of that statement becomes apparent when we realize that we cannot take life out of our food and replace it with chemicals, while serving the purpose for which it was intended.

CORRECTING THE MISTAKES OF GOD AND NATURE

Remember, the process that has just been described as taking place with wheat grain can actually be applied to every one of the foods that we enjoy in a modern, advanced society.

Not content to meddle in the processes of our plants and animals, our natural 'industrious' nature, has served to alter our water, our air and our whole natural way of life. But, has that stopped our progress? **No.**

We have become so pompous and proud of our new greatness that we've now set ourselves to the task (led by science) of correcting the 'mistakes' that Mother Nature and the Creator have made.

Science has now become so advanced that it feels justified (and the majority allow this kind of thinking) in assuming the authority to randomly destroy what it feels are worthless body organs.

The two obvious examples of this kind of thinking are the appendix and tonsils. These two organs have been systematically maligned by our medical industry (especially a few decades ago) as somehow foreign tissue dwelling within our bodies. In reality, both of these organs are now generally known to have a vital role in cleansing the body and helping to act as part of the body's alarm system. When they become totally overloaded with toxins, often they become inflamed. This is a signal from the body that something is wrong. So, what brilliant suggestions do we usually get in regard to these two organs? Medical professionals routinely suggest that we should cut these two organs from the body as they are 'unnecessary'. We suppose that the doctor will take the responsibility of these two organs and alert us if our body is in need of attention. Naturally, there will be a slight fee for this service.

There will also be a fee for the service of cutting these organs from your body...which, incredibly is a procedure that is usually recommended long before any signals from the body have even been sent to these organs. In other words, we don't even wait for the tonsils to become inflamed (warning us that we have a problem) before we slice them from our body.

Another way that science has determined to improve our lives is bizarrely related to our use of chemicals themselves. First, diseases are caused by chemicals; then the pharmaceutical industry takes the opportunity to create new drugs for every conceivable disease. There are literally hundreds of drugs for every single disease (and dozens of name brands of the same substances). There is a constant flow of new, improved, more powerful and extra strength drugs that are all basically the same substance, but each claiming to be some remarkable variation of the poison that preceded it. Whatever the claims, the end result is simply going to be more disease, in greater variety for a larger percent of the population. As long as we continue to willingly use the chemicals to both make ourselves sick and then try to cure the sickness, then we have to expect the chemical industry to continue to help us in our insane endeavors.

SILENCING THE BODY'S ALARMS

Before getting too far afield, we must return to our original premise that **disease is the exception, rather than the rule in nature.** Our basic starting point is simply this: The cause of all disease (major or minor) is toxicity which is obviously the end result of too much pollution, too many chemicals, a host of unnatural foods and an unnatural life-style. These 'causes' to our health problems are, in turn, effecting our ATTITUDE about our place in the natural environment.

We also know that the body has an alarm system to warn us when a serious situation is present, or when there is a threat to our health. This is a natural 'instinct', a gift from the Creator at the time of our making. One of the signals of this system is pain. Other symptoms (signals) are discomforts such as fatigue, stress, headaches or many others.

In our modern way of looking at things, instead of trying to determine why we are getting these signals from our bodies (or even attempting to eliminate the cause to our discomforts) we have chosen a lifestyle which promotes our putting chemicals into our system to suppress the warning signals. If your fire alarm went off in your house, would you cover it with a pillow or see where the smoke was coming from?

Our mass media is full of ads which most of us can recite by heart. If you have this type of ache or pain then you should take this medication. Nagging Arthritis? Take this! If that doesn't work, then try this EXTRA STRENGTH kind.

No advertiser presumes to tell you how to eliminate the cause, or even admit that there IS a cause. What they do tell you (with catchy phrases and jingles that work on your subconscious) is that their products can help you kill the pain...erase the symptom. These companies are out after one thing...money. They know that to make money, they have to either give the public what they want or convince you that what they have, is what you need. Some do a little of both, but if we didn't allow these companies to prey one us, by relinquishing control of our bodies to them, then they couldn't force their products down our throats.

We just don't pay close enough attention to what's happening. We've made ourselves good targets, but we can make ourselves difficult targets too. Most of these advertisements are even quick to include the disclaimer, "Temporary Relief." But, does this slow down our shopping spree, when the first sign of pain hits. No, in fact (knowing that this phrase is not given as an attempt at honesty on their parts) we do exactly what that phrase has intended for us to do. We rush to the corner market and stock up on the drugs to prevent us from running out when the doses we are taking wear off.

THE FIGURES SPEAK FOR THEMSELVES

In this section we've tried to briefly present a health sketch of our modern society for comparison with the primitive and 'backward' community in Hunza. Some people are probably saying that we're being too hard, or too dramatic in our estimation of our current situation. But, we say that when the ship is sinking, the sailors do not try to think of a nice way to tell you that 'the ship is sinking.' There is no reason to try and be cool and calm, when disaster is literally staring us in the face.

We hope that the picture that was earlier drawn of Hunza is enough of an illustration for you to compare what you know about our own society. Now, what we'd like to do is conclude this comparison with some official statistics and estimates from related authorities, that are supposed to help justify the belief that modern technology and medical science have achieved wonders.

Seen with an open mind, using the voice of Common Sense to guide you, we believe that the figures presented will be able to speak for themselves on how we feel.

PREVALENCE OF MAJOR DISEASES, PHYSICAL AND MENTAL DISORDERS IN THE UNITED STATES

Heart or blood vessel disease
     41,300,000
     Statistics by American Heart Association
Cancer (under medical care in 1970's)   10,000,000
     Statistics by American Cancer Society
Lung Disease   47,000,000
     (Chronic respiratory disease)
     e.g. Asthma, Bronchitis, Emphysema,
     Statistics by American Lung Association
Arthritis   35,000,000
     Statistics by Arthritis Foundation
Liver Disease (Including Cirrhosis)   25,000,000
     Estimated by independent body
Kidney Disease
13,000,000
     Statistics by National Kidney Foundation
Mental Disorder   32,000,000
     (people in need of some mental health service)
Herpes   20,000,000
     (Simple type II)
     Estimated by Federal Centers for
     Disease Control
Diabetes   10,700,000
     Statistics by American Diabetes Association
Migraine   16,000,000
     Estimate from the Migraine Foundation
     from 14 to 18 million
Problem Drinker   13,000,000
     Estimated by National Institute on

Alcohol Abuse and Alcoholism
Mentally Retarded   2,000,000
Statistics by Association for Retarded Citizens
Obesity   80,000,000
(Individuals facing weight problems)
Estimated from various independent bodies

Note:The adult population for these figures is estimated to be about 142 million. These figures have been recently updated in some cases.

The statistical and projected figures that we presented do not include minor diseases and discomforts, the list of which would be a book in itself. These 'minor' afflictions would include such things as indigestion, constipation, insomnia, colds, flu, and others. They also do not include the newest scourge on modern society, AIDS or the projected numbers of non-medical drug users. The number of those who have ever used different drugs is detailed below:

Marijuana, Hashish:	54,800,000
Inhalants:	12,700,000
Hallucinogens:	15,800,000
P.C.P.:	8,200,000
Cocaine:	15,100,000
Heroin:	2,600,000
Stimulants:	13,900,000
Sedatives:	11,100,000
Tranquilizers:	9,800,000

These estimates, again, are probably quite low since they are based on a 1979 National survey on drug abuse conducted by the U.S. Department Of Health and Human Services. However, they are still accurate as a comparison (some will be slightly more or less), and are shocking when your learn that the total number of people who ever used marijuana (for instance) exceeds 54,000,000 even at the time of this outdated survey. However, this may be misleading since it cannot be disassociated from qualifying factors such as the percentage of individuals who have used drugs once only or abuse more than one type of drug. Whatever way these statistics are interpreted they still indicate the serious health problems (both emotional and physical) which are caused by or a result of drug abuse.

This information and the chart that preceded it, are presented in the hope that certain questions will be brought to your mind. **Am I healthy? Are my loved ones healthy ?** And, most importantly, **who are the healthy people in the U.S.,** and **WHY ARE THEY HEALTHY?**

When we allow ourselves to think about these things, and ask our inner voice for answers to these questions, other, more personal questions will be inspired, such as (we hope): Isn't it time to give some serious thought to the condition of your personal health and the health of your loved ones?

CHAPTER NINE

THE FACTS ABOUT REAL HUMAN FOOD

Have you ever thought about how amazing all those "primitive cultures" are to have been able to find out the medicinal value of plants without any scientific testing? The fact of the matter is that NO new value has ever been discovered by, so called 'modern science" that the 'primitive cultures didn't already know about. Modern Science has really not done anything for humanity in regard to health and medicine. We hear praise for 'discoveries' such as penicillin or aspirin, but the Native Americans already were using these things thousands of years before Columbus invaded their shores. In truth, most Modern Discoveries have been stolen from some primitive people, who was using the medicine in a harmonious way with the laws of nature. In addition, all the vitamins, minerals and other nutritional elements that scientists have based their nutritional standards on were originally "discovered" to be present in natural foods. This may seem like a simple statement but we believe it is one that needs to be made. Every nutrient, vitamins A through Z and all the rest that have ever been categorized, are only a fraction of the elements that will ever be found in real live food. But, THEY'RE ALREADY IN THE

FOOD! They've always been there, and would always BE there, if we hadn't worked so hard to change things.

Additionally, all the nutritional elements that are present in the basic food items can be found in the by-products and variations of these basic foods, but the textures, combinations and ratios of these will be different. This means that dairy products, for instance, will be found to contain the same basic elements of human nutrition because animals eat a variety of the same natural foods and the milk that they produce will certainly possess many of the same nutrients that the original food did. Similarly, the flesh of a herbivore contains the same elements that are in fresh natural food (but, again in an altered texture, combination and ratio), as the animal has been feeding his body on these same foods. This does not mean that milk or meat is the same as natural human food! There are differences between the elements in an animal's flesh or what an animal produces as a by-product, and what was originally used as the building blocks to create the animal. If we truly believed that we became the EXACT elements that we ate, then the only real flesh we should eat (by this logic) would be HUMAN flesh. Obviously, cannibalism is NOT the answer. The answer is to get our nutrition FROM THE SOURCE, as was intended by nature. The trickle down theory does not hold true in the economics of human nourishment.

In analyzing the relative nutritional values of various foods It will be easier for us to separate our conventional foods into three broad categories: dairy products (anything made of milk), animal flesh (including poultry, eggs, fish and other seafood), and natural human food (anything that grows from the ground such as fruits, nuts, vegetables, green leaves and seeds). Of course there are numerous 'created' foods' that are almost solely chemical in composition (instant this and lite that), but most of these fall into one of the above categories. Our purpose here is to logically prove which of these broad categories of foods are NOT fit for human consumption and in that way demonstrate which of these categories are "proper human food."

To discuss dairy products sufficiently, it will be enough to discuss only milk, as this is the basic material of all dairy products. In this case, to determine what is proper for human consumption, we shall examine the laws of nature and see what the purpose was in producing the product in the first place. In this way we'll see that milk (other than mother's milk) is not fit for humans.

In scripture, when creation took place, each creature was commanded to produce offspring 'after its own kind'. Each animal and plant, thereby was directed to follow its own, SPECIALIZED COURSE of growth in life.

In regards to mammals, each mammal has is own 'life span', purpose and developmental process. Dogs develop according to the rules of dogs, cats according to the rules of cats and cows, according to their own set of natural laws (each being harmonious with the other's).

Cow's milk, then, was produced specifically for baby cows to grow on. It is as precisely formulated toward that goal, as human's milk is made to meet the nutritional needs and requirements of human babies. These nutritional needs are unique and distinct. It is not logical, therefore, to assume that all milk is the same. And, if we examine milk (in general) even a little more closely, we will see just how true this statement is.

Rabbit's milk has, for instance, ten times the amount of protein that human milk has. A baby rabbit must double its size during the first week of life if it is going to survive. Seal's milk is forty percent fat, because a seal needs to develop a good layer of insulation for protection against cold waters. Human milk contains lactalbumin, which furnishes the baby with important amino acids. Cow's milk contains none of this material, but is high in a mucousy material called casein. This milk has everything that a baby cow will need to grow at the proper pace, according to its own physiological needs. Casein is not good for humans, and is also used in making glue.

Interestingly, not only have we been brainwashed to substitute cow's milk for human's in the care of infants, but science (not too long ago) also decided that human milk was actually inferior to a "balanced simulation" that technology had come up with. They had corrected another "mistake" of nature and business interests benefited as millions of mothers believed that the newly created baby powders and chemical concoctions were actually superior to the "inferior mixture" that nature had taken eons to come up with.

Today, we know that there is nothing so healthy for baby humans as mother's own milk. Practically every human mother who is able to, goes out of her way (even in a modern society where it is difficult) to furnish her children with the nutrition they need for growth.

Unfortunately, the same kind of logic that almost put mother's breast out of business is exactly the same kind that has given rise to the entire dairy industry. Natural protein isn't any good (they say) use cheese, and so on. there has been such a brainwashing about milk that now, to prove that something is natural, the dairy industry has gotten other advertisers to say, "contains real milk." The truth is that milk products (this includes, so called NON-fat ones) are so high in fat that long time users greatly increase the risks of many kinds of diseases associated with this kind of poison. So much for dairy products; let's move on to the meat industry

ANIMAL FLESH

Based on the laws of nature, the food of any creature will also correspond to its physical structure. The general body shape of an animal, as well as specifics about physical characteristics such as the mouth and jaw, teeth and digestive system will tell us what his function is on the food chain.

In the science of biology, the vertebrates are usually classified into three groups. These are the meat eaters, the grass and leaf eaters and the fruit and nut eaters. Below we have included a chart that takes into account some of the physical characteristics of each to show what group humans should belong to. For convenience sake and easier identification we've created a new subgroup called "vegetarian animals" that combines the grass and leaf eaters and the fruit and nut eaters, since humans fall into both categories.

MEAT EATERS	VEGETARIAN ANIMALS	HUMANS
Have claws	No claws	No claws
Have elongated sharp teeth and powerful jaws that move essentially up & down.	No elongated sharp front teeth. Jaws move side ways.	No elongated sharp front teeth. Jaws move side ways.
Small glands in the mouth.	Large glands in the mouth.	Large glands in the mouth.

Continued on next page

Acid saliva with no enzyme ptyalin.	Acid saliva with much enzyme ptyalin	Acid saliva with much enzyme ptyalin
No molar teeth.	Many molars.	Many molars.
Strong stomach acid.	Weak acid in stomach.	Weak acid in stomach.
Intestinal tract about 3 times the body length.	Intestines about 10 times the body length.	Intestines about 10 times the body length..
Perspires through the tongue and no pores on the skin.	Perspires with aid of sweat glands with millions of pores on the skin.	Perspires with aid of sweat glands with millions of pores on the skin

With this chart in mind, how should we interpret these facts? A long and powerful jaw that moves only up and down, teeth that are sharp in front and claws are all characteristics that would prove valuable for meat eaters that must catch, hold, pierce, kill and tear the flesh of their prey. The vegetarian animal needs many molars that move sideways to aid in grinding. They need no elongated, sharp front teeth, except perhaps two for protection.

How should we interpret the facts derived from this chart? Even as Scripture said that all creatures were created 'according to their own kind', Humans have certain characteristics that classify them among one of these groups. Carnivores (meat eaters) have the equipment that they need to perform their function on the food chain. To kill and tear flesh, they must have sharp claws and teeth.   The vegetarian animal needs many molars that move sideways for grinding, but do not need elongated front teeth nor powerful claws.

The digestive system of a carnivore has stomach acids that are up to ten times stronger than the vegetarians and a short intestinal tract. This is due to the fact that animal flesh decays rapidly and would have a chance to produce poisons if it were not digested quickly and allowed to stay in the intestines for a long time. Yes, the Creator's plan was well laid. He made room for the meat eaters to help keep the sick and wounded numbers low. The strong saliva is an example of how these creatures are cared for.

The vegetarian animal, on the other hand, has saliva which is high in alkaline and contains plenty of enzyme ptyalin. This is appropriate for digesting the natural sugars and starches found in all natural foods, and would not have any logical effect on the digestion of animal flesh (which it doesn't). Vegetarians also have long and sophisticated intestines and colon systems, equipped to handle the process of breaking down the natural foods (fruits, nuts, vegetables, leaves and seeds) which involves by necessity a process of fermentation. This process uses bacteria to break down the food fibers and complete the digestion process.

There is nothing in the human physiology, eating mechanism, digestive tract or other characteristics that would justify the conclusion that we are 'naturally' meat eating creatures. All of our organs and digestive components are identical to those of the vegetarian animal. We have very little in common with carnivores (except for an obnoxious aggressiveness). Wouldn't it be logical for us to assume that we are vegetarians and NOT meat eaters?

Many researchers make much out of our aggressive behavior as a point to justify humans in the carnivorous category. However, close scrutiny by our most thoughtful investigators indicates that we are aggressive BECAUSE we eat meat, not the other way around. In other words, eating flesh has a bad side-effect on human behavior (one of many) and this is that it makes us a little crazy.

If we compare those societies on earth who are vegetarian with those who eat meat as a staple, then we will see a direct correspondence between the diet and the level of aggression. The people who eat little or NO meat are the most peaceful. The communities of Hunza and those others we've mentioned as Super Healthy are well known for being crime free.

NATURAL HUMAN FOOD

A quick analysis of the evidence shows us that animal milk (dairy products) and meat are not natural human food.   And, if we examine further we see that biologically, functionally and in all other ways WE ARE NOT MEAT EATERS, WE ARE VEGETARIANS! Natural Human Nutrition, therefore is the living foods; fruits, nuts, grains, vegetables and green leaves that our ancestors (and our current-day, peaceful and healthy counterparts) consumed.

It is essential to note that we draw these conclusions not only based upon the laws of man, but by examining the evidence in regard to the laws of Nature.

We didn't begin this chapter by asking, "What does Science tell us," because, we understand that today the laws of science and the laws of nature are serving two different masters. Modern-day Science is so involved in serving the corporate structure that it now exists outside our world of realities. But, regardless of how hard they try to disguise the fact, there will come a time when it will become obvious to all that we cannot take one more step on our current road without signing our own death warrant. When our FINAL DESTRUCTION is imminent, then all the politicians and scientists will have to come back and try to erase the effects of their deviations from the laws of nature. Let's hope that it won't be too late.

Some examples of the urgency of changing our habits have been seen in the news lately with headlines about the Ozone Layer. After years of producing hazardous chemicals, scientists have discovered that there IS a breaking point for our carelessness. The phenomenon has reached the level where it COULD be too late.

So now we are getting together in world-wide conferences to find a way to avoid total destruction that we once thought could come only in nuclear war. And, speaking of nuclear war, that brings to mind another fine example of how technology has gotten out of hand. We've produced so many nuclear weapons that we have the power to destroy the earth dozens of times over. And, if we don't kill everything and everybody with the initial blasts, then their will be enough debris left flying in the air to poison us later, or to change the atmosphere (Nuclear Winter) by blocking out the sun for decades.

Interestingly, we began to look closely at the Nuclear Question at a time when we were creating OTHER weapons of war that would haunt us for generations. Here, we are talking about Agent Orange, a plant killing agent that was used heavily during the Viet Nam war. The Idea behind Agent Orange was to destroy vegetation without doing harm to the people (but giving the Vietnamese army fewer places to hide). Not only did this deadly chemical KILL MANY men, women and children by poisoning, but it continues to kill, maim and torture hundreds and thousands of American Servicemen who came into contact with it during their service to our country.   These lessons, sometimes are made sadly graphic, as is the case with Agent Orange. For, it was recently learned that the son of the general who ordered all the spraying of this chemical, later contracted cancer and died AS A DIRECT RESULT OF HIS CONTACT WITH THIS CHEMICAL.

This, we believe will be the case with ALL businesses who do not heed the laws of nature. Every Giant Industry, no matter how much money they have, will be subject to the same economic laws of Life And Health as the rest of us. No amount of complicated knowledge (unused) will protect Science from destruction it creates for itself by trying to by-pass the simplicity of the natural order. No level of cash flow will prevent the ultimate collapse of the corporate structure that proceeds in opposition to the force of life.

Ironically, when we examine the laws of nature and draw our conclusions from these laws, we are only doing what science USED to do, and should still be doing. All the great scientific discoveries, including those of Newton, Copernicus, Galileo or Einstein (with his discovery of the tremendous power of the atom), are based upon observations of the natural laws. True science is (and has always been, regardless of what Scientists want us to believe) nothing more than gaining a knowledge of the laws that the Creator gave us to abide by. These laws govern the whole universe, and our task as natural seekers, is to learn how to utilize our new knowledge and understanding of the natural order, for the benefit of all creation.

In light of our new knowledge about the woes that humans have placed themselves and the earth in, we should understand that business is not going to change their focus (which is to make money at any cost). What we must do (those of us who want to follow the laws of the Creator) is demonstrate to business how it is in their best interest to follow these same laws.

Remember, it is another very simple principle that motivates business. The law of Supply and Demand is one that is based upon a model of the Creator's. Our responsibility is to make our demands more in line with the natural laws. We shouldn't just accept what is offered. Those who want to supply us (business) will profit ONLY when they offer products and goods that coincide with our desires.

We should honor and respect those scientists who still put human well-being and the welfare of the whole earth before the interests of business by drawing impartial conclusions from their observations.
The purity and value of science CAN be preserved. Human life CAN be improved! People CAN make a "living" out of offering life over death and disease.

This does not mean that we should be looking for more comforts and conveniences to take us further away from the natural order. We can easily see, by using the people of Hunza as an example, that the more gadgets and comforts that we pile up will not mean better health for us or a happier, longer life.

THE THEORY OF SUPPLEMENTS

If we could eat nothing but live, natural food, grown in a fertile soil, and we were able to adhere to the Ten Commandments of Health, we definitely would not have to experience any disease (major or minor). We might also, as the people of Hunza, not know what headaches, stress, back pain or allergies are.

We say "might", because our environment is not as clean as theirs and our genes are not as healthy as those produced under their conditions. But, IF we could change some major things about our current conditions, then it is certain that our overall health could be increased ten fold.

Unfortunately, we know that we DON'T get the quality of food that we should. In fact, we consume a lot of empty junk foods and, further, the live, natural foods that we DO eat have lost a good deal of their nutritional value if not all.

Why has there been such a change in our produce? There are a number of reasons, really, but mainly it is due to chemicals. These chemicals come in the form of fertilizers and pesticides that we have been dumping into our soil and spraying onto our plants for many decades. These SOIL DESTROYING CHEMICALS have become so abundant that they now are found throughout the natural environment. There is not a single part of the natural system that has been able to remain immune. Even as waters are evaporated into the air and are returned to the earth in the form of rain, these same chemicals (sometimes in even worse forms than originally found) come back to haunt the farmlands as a new source of destruction...Acid Rain!

Actually, Acid Rain has been washing into our soils since the Industrial Revolution, but we didn't know about it until recently. We will explain the phenomenon of Acid Rain in a later chapter, but here, suffice it to say that even our 'natural' food, does not have the quality OR the potency that good, healthful and natural food SHOULD have.

The Theory of Supplements is that scientists have studied natural food in its highest potency and quality and determined (according to knowledge about the human physiology) that there is a great potential for nutritional shortages. To replenish these shortages these same scientists have come up with different formulas to replenish what we lack in our diet, or what our technologically produced foods can no longer give to us.

There are thousands of different pills, capsules, extracts and various combinations of these, that are produced everyday. We also know that millions of people take them.

Unfortunately, our enslavement by a modern life-style has restricted our access to the fuels (live, organically grown foods) that our bodies needs. These foods would obviously be EVEN BETTER if they were produced in a fertile, natural, unpolluted soil and environment. For this reason (understandably) many of us have taken to the practice of trying to give our body the nourishment it requires in some other form. This basic, instinctual drive on our part has been instrumental in creating supplements.

A funny new twist to the question of supplements has been seen in the media lately. This is when certain doctors have come forward with indignant tones in their voices to tell us that vitamins and other supplements are worthless. And, that all those health food 'nuts' who are trying to get you to take vitamins are lying to you. Some of these same doctors even go so far as to proclaim that 'every vitamin you need, you will get from a balanced diet.' Probably, the phrase 'a balanced diet' includes eating daily amounts of meat, dairy products and may even include a cup or two of coffee and a daily, alcoholic drink or two. Then, they add insult to injury and make these comments in a way that suggests that we, 'the common folk' are not quite smart enough to take care of ourselves, that we should rely upon 'the knowledgeable' (doctors and scientists) to do our health thinking for us.

Unfortunately, what they don't tell you is to get a balanced diet, you must eat only natural foods and high quality nutrition from real ORGANICALLY cultivated (fertile and unpolluted) soil. Another 'omitted' piece of information is that most of produce, fruits, nuts and grains that we get on our supermarket shelves are practically devoid of the nutrition that EVEN these people KNOW we need.

Certainly, if they wanted to truly help us, they'd recommend that we eat live food. But, so far, none who've made it to national television has had this approach.

Trying our best to unravel the confused mysteries of supplements, we've come up with what we believe is the best advice possible. Because your foods are probably NOT giving your body all that it needs, then you MIGHT want to try supplements (vitamins, minerals, etc.) as a way to counteract a known deficiency. However, be forewarned, even within the realm of supplements there is the danger that you are not getting what you THINK you are getting. Do not use vitamins, for instance, that are not produced by something akin to natural means, using as little processing as possible. You also want to make CERTAIN that you are not merely pumping into your body WORSE chemicals than the ones you think you're supplying yourself with.

Vitamin C, for example, can be produced in a number of ways for tablets and capsules. Make sure that you get your C from a natural source, such as Rose Hips or acerola. Chemical creations that are supposed to 'resemble' vitamins in every way ARE NOT THE SAME AS THE ONES PRODUCED BY NATURE.

Also, make sure that the fillers you are getting with your supplements are not more empty chemicals,but are indeed natural foods themselves. In short, the more pure and close to NATURAL that your supplements are, the better they will be for you in the long run.

CHAPTER TEN

LET NATURAL FOOD BE YOUR MEDICINE

If what you've read so far makes sense, then you'll agree that food can and should be categorized in ONLY two ways, either the food is pure and natural (with all its health giving qualities) or it isn't.

This simple distinction holds true, especially in modern times. To take this one step further would be to say that the two ways of categorizing are 1) according to the level of health hazard, or 2) according to their level of benefit to the human body. These are the two categories that we'll use in this chapter.

If we take this one step further, we can see that in both cases (being harmful or healthful) foods could be categorized more precisely by their LEVEL of toxicity or healthfulness. At this point we will present our OWN distinctions, according to these categories. We realize that some of our readers may not approve of the way that we view a 'specific' item. THAT'S PERFECTLY ALRIGHT.

We are not presenting these distinctions to solicit agreement or win arguments. We merely want you to have a clear understanding of our perspective. Our conclusions are not based upon extensive research or long term studies, but are arrived at according to our own, limited studies and our knowledge which comes from experience.

With this in mind, let's organize foods that are hazardous into two separate sub-categories. One would be those foods that are THE MOST HAZARDOUS to human health. This sub-category includes anything having chemicals (additives, preservatives,artificial colors and many others) fat, red meat, sugar, white flour, coffee, alcohol, dairy products, soda drinks.

Our second 'sub-category' of hazardous foods are those similar,but less refined (less chemicalized or 'less hazardous') items such as some white meats (skinless chicken white meat or fish), unrefined sugar, white rice, white cheese (those with very low fat content), foods and vegetables that have been processed only for packaging.

Now that we have a clearer understanding of what we mean by Hazardous foods, let's look at what we consider HEALTHFUL (revitalizing and healing). Under this broad heading we can again divide our foods into two sub-groups. The first sub-group consists of cooked and frozen vegetables, all living foods (such as vegetables, nuts, fruits, grains etc.) that have been produced with the aid of chemical fertilizers (so called commercially grown). These are foods that have been produced on an inferior land (we will discuss the subject of inferior versus fertile land in another chapter).

We make this statement with a bit of hesitation, since we don't want anyone to get the idea that we support chemicals in any form. On the other hand we must consider the following point. In the U.S. today, MOST of our produce comes from commercially grown sources. This is generally the ONLY food that is available to us. Secondly, it APPEARS that the value we receive from the circumstance of eating LIVE FOOD (even commercially grown) makes these foods better than those in the category of Hazardous Foods although we DO NOT APPROVE IT AS 100% LIVE FOOD. Obviously, we must point out (again) that these chemicals are NOT NECESSARY and only serve to harm the overall nutritional as well as the healing qualities of the food. Also, the more chemicals that are added, the worse (and therefore NEGATIVE) the balance becomes. If, for instance, we start to add pesticides to the soil, and/or the plants, and/or the fruits and vegetables themselves then it just isn't worth it any longer. And, when high quantities of nitrogen and oxygen are pumped into the soil for the sole purpose of making our fruits bigger (but not better), then, again we qualify our original statement about this category.

Finally, we come to the sub-category of PURE, NATURAL, HUMAN FOODS. These are obviously going to be THE BEST. They are grown in unpolluted soil, organically, with the cleanest water and most natural methods available. This food (**with one exception**) we can compare to that which nourishes the people of Hunza and Vilcabamba. It can also be sub-divided into various levels of purity. And, is best when eaten, fresh and raw, as was intended by nature. The **exception** (of our commercially grown food versus the food grown in super healthy communities of Hunza and Vilcabamba) is based on the knowledge that the food of Hunza or Vilcabamba comes from an **extremely fertile soil.** It has been observed that all the places we've just mentioned are located in high altitudes and thy grow their food on land which is unbelievably rich in minerals. There is speculation that all such lands are either close to present volcanic mountain regions OR that the soil is rich in volcanic residue due to past volcanic activity. This is not usually the case with commercial growing enterprises.

Now, let's examine a constant battle that our bodies are waging in regard to the categories that we've just outlined. The poisons from the first three categories outlined. The poisons from the first three categories above, gradually are being pumped into our bodies clogging our digestive systems and preventing the nourishing elements from reaching our organs. The period of time that is necessary for any one food to do its ultimate damage depends on its own toxic strength and the present ability of our bodies to compensate for these ill-effects. It also depends how much and how often live food (if any) we are giving our systems, and the healing qualities of the food. We'll explain that in a moment.

Another important point must be made here: the factor of youthfulness affects the ability of our bodies to expel the toxins we consume. This is only natural. Broken bones heal more slowly when we are older, even if we are getting proper nutrition. On the other hand, in a place like Hunza, a broken bone is an extreme rarity, since even the bodies of the very old in Hunza are better able to cope with stress than those of most young people in a modern civilization. So, Age and other factors (such as cosmetics and dirty air) are considerations, but are secondary to the fact that most of the toxins (and the most damaging) are put into our bodies along with the food we eat. Our bodies are expecting to be nourished and healed by foods, so it's a 'dirty trick' when that doesn't happen.

So, although we are subjected to toxic materials in a number of ways in a modern society, the main factor that could throw the balance from ill-health to health (or vice versa) is the ratio of toxic intake to the clean, natural, healing foods.

As an example of what we are saying we have only to examine those individuals in our own society whose testimonials you have read. These people surely take toxic materials into their systems (through air, water or other pollutants) but their intake/ratio of natural human foods versus the unnatural foods and toxic wastes is so high (varying from individual to individual) that their bodies are in a constant state of cleansing. Gradually this process has helped them expel the toxins in their systems and is the key factor in their health. This same ratio, we must point out, should be an individual goal in terms of our own health as well as toward the world in general. If we clean up more pollution than we make, then cleansing on a global basis can begin. In both cases, the old saying applies, "two steps forward and one step back and you're making progress."

THE CLEANSING PROCESS AND THE SCIENCE OF NATURAL HEALING

Let us clear one important point before we go any further. In natural healing the process that your body has to go through to heal your ills, is the same process that your body needs in a healthy condition to maintain health, vitality, energy and preserve all the physical, sexual and mental faculties. In other words, the requirements that will keep your body DISEASE FREE, VITAL and HEALTHY (like people of Hunza and Vilcabamba) are the same requirements that your body needs to rid itself from disease and ill-health. This is unlike our conventional medicine and therefore might not be very clear to some of you. We are lead to believe that our bodies requirement in health is different from when we are in ill-health. When we are in ill-health we should go to the doctor and we should take a variety of medicine on doctors prescription and once we are back to health we are also back to the old way - offending foods and unhealthy lifestyle until we are back to disease. It is a common knowledge that you can not stay on one medication for long because of its adverse side effects. If the symptoms of disease do not go away you should change medication and if it did "relieve" you from the symptoms of the disease (not the disease itself) then you should stop medication and go back to your old offending foods and unhealthy lifestyle. What is this telling us. It is telling us that medication is a temporary thing and it is worse than your offending foods that caused you the disease in the first place.

In natural healing it is just the opposite. The process or the medication which is required, while you are in ill-health is the same as what you need for prevention, energy and vitality when you are in perfect health.

WHAT IS NATURAL HEALING OR PREVENTION?

The ability of the body to prevent disease and keep itself in youthful a state or heal itself from disease is mainly dependent upon two factors.

a) The cleanliness of your digestive tract (where the food is being processed, analyzed and required nutrition absorbed).

b) The nutrition (the fuel which contains all required nutritional elements) that is provided to your body to function upon.

When we talk about cleanliness of our digestive tract we should bear in mind two important things. First, that under any living conditions (as healthy as Hunza or unhealthy like ours) the human body accumulates some waste and unwanted substances. This accumulation of waste slows down our body's effeciency which we label as "aging". Second and equally important is that once your digestive tract is relatively filled with these poisonous materials it is then, passed through the circulatory system to the other parts of the body. Usually it is imposed to different organs of the body starting with the weakest one and then the second weakest one. This is how discomfort and different diseases set in the joints, kidney, liver, heart or the others.

In ideal healthy, living conditions (like Hunza or Vilcabamba) the accumulation of waste is so minute and therefore the body's slowing down is minimal.

In unhealthy conventional living conditions (like industrial Countries including United States) the accumulation of waste is out of proportion. Therefore, the aging comes not only with a considerable slowing down but also brings a host of disease and ailments. Regardless of what others might tell you, we will slow down in all areas, the older we get. THIS DOESN'T MEAN THAT WE SHOULD EXPECT DEBILITATION AND DISEASE WHEN WE GET OLDER. FAR FROM IT, if we can maintain relatively healthy living conditions.

But, it is only logical to assume that we will not have the EXACT same capabilities when old, that we did when young. But there should not be a dramatic difference either.

Obviously when we grow we change. Older runners slow down, but they can usually run farther (endurance increases) that is why we have young sprinters and older long distance runners.

When we grow, we gain experience and get wiser while the young gets new advanced knowledge. That is just the way that it is.

There is nothing wrong with aging. It is natural and we need to accept change as part of the natural order of things

Therefore, the natural healing will work on the young the same way as it will work on the elderly, except for time. Because when we age (especially with our very unhealthy conventional food) we accumulate a considerable amount of waste. Therefore, it takes much much longer to clean out when we are older. The natural healing should work the same way as you are in ill-health or in perfect health. If you are in ill-health it will work as a healing process and while healthy it will work as a preventive process maintaining your health vitality and preserving your physical, sexual, and mental capabilities.

HOW NATURAL HEALING WORKS

For your body to administer the Natural Healing process it is necessary to provide your body with the proper tool in order a) to clean the system b) obtain the required nutritional elements for healing and/or prevention.

The first and foremost tool is your food (nutrition). You must provide your body with a quality of food (nutrition) that will provide the cleansing material (fiber) and High Quality Nutrition which is the base for all required elements in a quality and potency that will provide the healing process as well as the prevention if you are in a healthy condition.

Obviously the food (nutrition) you provide your body is the first and foremost tool but all the other Ten Commandments of Hunza health should be observed in order to improve and enhance the results.

HEALING BY MODERN MEDICAL SCIENCE

The solutions that modern medical science have come up with are (at the same time) typical and incredible. They are typical because they respond first to the the money incentives and lastly to the needs of the people in question. They are incredible because, as a society, we continue to let these people prey on us with their 'experimental mentality'. Their answer to combat the fact that we've filled our bodies, for many decades full of toxins is to prescribe 'more toxins'. First, they prepare our bodies to combat the symptoms by giving us 'symptom suppressants' (usually this means pain killers). In our understanding the symptoms (usually aches and pains) are the language that our bodies talk to us with and tell us that something is wrong inside. Now our conventional medical science instead of listening to the body's talk and do something about it they suppress it. Then later, when real disease sets in, we are bombarded with a new barrage of medicines. Some of this medication is merely added to our bodies so that new testing can be completed. How many people do you know who've had radioactive dye pumped into their veins so that some kind of x-ray examination could be performed?

And, if all the prescriptions to prevent disease don't do the trick and the initial tests turn up nothing (which they seldom do) then the final 'search and destroy mission' is to go in and cut out the offending organs or the entire warning system. Looked at in this light, isn't it incredible that we've allowed the control of our own health to get so out of hand?

And, isn't it amazing that when a group of people band together to give us the health truth they are usually marked as crackpots, by the same self-proclaimed geniuses who recommend cutting out parts of your body for preventative purposes. This is what has happened, we believe, to the naturopathic healers. They have gotten a 'bad name' from doctors and scientists because they were honest enough to stand up for natural health. But, you can judge for yourself.

The science of natural healing rightly reports that man-made chemicals only add to the natural problems by contributing to the quantity of toxins in our systems. We believe that the body must be given the proper equipment (fuel) to facilitate its own healings. Even an OLD body can run at top efficiency, just as an old car can run well. But like the vintage model vehicle, you only get as good as you give. You've got to take care of your car if you expect it to last a while. The same is true of your body. The validity of these beliefs are proven by the success of natural treatments.

All along we have been using the word "cleansing" and factually this is the process that our bodies must go through to achieve good health. This is a chain reaction condition, that begins the first day that the amount of high quality nutrition you eat, is greater than the amount of unnatural, toxic food. When natural high quality foods are given to the system in a high ratio, then the result will be healing. Cleansing your body of poisons will create gradual improvement and proper function of the various organs of the body. These ever improving organs will, in turn, affect the health of one another, giving direction and gradual improvement to the general health of the whole body. When the body is KEPT in a state of healing and cleansing, then it is only logical to assume that the overall health will be superior FOR A LONGER TIME. A healthy young person (in other words) creates the right circumstances for the healthy OLD PERSON that they will develop into at a later time in life.

Certainly, there are a number of factors involved. Old people in our country are not given the opportunity to be healthful and vigorous. Often, the elder members of families or businesses are forced out of the system that sustains them. We put our old folks into nursing homes and make retirement mandatory at a very young age. With plastic pumps and tubes science has even been able to ward off death in some cases. But, this is a question of quality versus quantity. Who wants to live attached to a machine, dependent on air hoses and kidney dialysis for survival? Is that living? Not in our opinion. And, what is the most important element that can make A BIG difference? The food and the nutrition that you take.

All the natural foods are gifted with effective cleansing agents and healing powers. Some of these foods, obviously, have stronger cleansing properties and will rid the body more quickly of toxic materials. These food items are the ones considered to have a stronger healing power. This (you might recall) is especially true of those foods that are grown In extremely clean, natural soils. This healing power, intrinsic in natural human foods, we call "the MEDICINE in natural foods." It is as if real, natural human food has a mind or intent to keep our bodies healthy. If we allow these natural healing agents to do the job they were intended for, then we will be fine. But, most of us "Kill the medicine" before it's allowed to help us. We kill our natural food's powers with chemicals, by cooking, or sometimes we destroy him before he is allowed to grow to help us (by polluting the soil, water etc.).

To really feel this "powerful medicine" our sincere advice is to stick closely to our   Hunza Health recommendations as long as you can, and even better make the whole of "Ten Commandments For Health" your lifestyle. Naturally, if you eat a higher ratio of cleansing agents with healing powers, the health results should come much faster and be more amazing.

The SCRIPTURE tell us that we will 'reap what we sow'. We add that not only will we reap what we sow, but we must eat what we reap as well. And, if we reap polluted, chemicalized foods, then we cannot expect to benefit from our harvest. At least, we cannot expect to benefit in the way, or to the extent that the CREATOR intended.

CHAPTER ELEVEN

THE DOCTOR IN YOUR BODY

As we have seen, the subject of the Human Body is a complex and beautiful one. When we consider every facet of influence that goes into making up the total individual, we can certainly agree with the words of Shakespeare, "What a piece of work is man! "

Although, we've made a big mess of things in the past few hundred years we believe that humans DO possess a "GOODNESS" (which comes from god-ness) that will enable us to rise to our challenges. At the heart of this God-like quality, as we've stated, is that part of us that is our direct link with the Creator, our inner voice or Common Sense. The search for the Ultimate Truth in regards to Ultimate Health, has been our goal.

There is a tremendous amount of knowledge that can still be learned in relation to the natural functioning of the human body. Health subjects are as large as the entire scope of evolution or as small as studying an individual cell. But, to take care of your own body all you must really know are a few simple facts. This 'simplicity', we believe is part of the beauty of the Creator's original plan. Those who want to complicate matters with 'new, startling discoveries' are only serving their own special interests.

Over the centuries the people who have been "practicing medicine" have been creating credibility for themselves by shrouding all of their knowledge in mystery. This type of tactic is part of a series of strategies that the people of "modern" medical science" use to maintain a position of authority over the general population. They simply want you to give them the responsibility for your health and not ask any questions. If you DO ask questions, then you are regarded with contempt or are confused with specialized language. There is a story of a man who went to a physician because of a pain he was having in his stomach. After hours of testing (mostly performed by nurses and assistant office staff) the physician came into the examination room with his prescription tablet and a professional air of authority. "It doesn't look serious," he told the patient. "Try this medication for a few days. If the pain doesn't go away, then please come back."

"What are you giving me?" The patient asked, throwing the physician off his guard for a moment.

"It's very complicated," started the physician, after regaining his composure. "You see, in some patients, the over stimulation of the intestines creates a colic-like condition within the stomach, causing the salivary and other glands to over-secrete gastric juices, which, in turn raises the level of hydrochloric acid and the enzyme pepsin in the digestive tract. This medication will help to alleviate the problem."

The patient took the script from the doctor and looked it over. What the physician didn't know was that the patient was ALSO a doctor who was merely looking for a second opinion. "So, in other words," said the patient with mischievous glint in his eye, "I have gas and you're giving me antacids?"

The truth of the matter is that a physician has NO healing powers when it comes to any other persons body. As we've already stated, science has done wondrous things in regards to individual cases. People who are born without hips or other bones, can be made to walk with inserts that science has devised. Those who lose a limb in an accident, can now get mechanical help in the form of prosthetics (man-made limbs). We are, as a species even able to take parts of eyes from those killed in accidents and give them to blind people to restore sight. But, these are all examples of technological manipulation of the body. We still cannot truly heal OR make a person healthy.

These abilities are really "instinctive gifts" and take place within your own body. This healing power will activate from natural food which is also the necessary fuel for the body to function at 100% efficiency. If you put the wrong fuel (unnatural foods) in your system, your body will have a double fight on its hands. First you will be constantly increasing the level of toxic wastes that will be going in (and needing to be cleaned out), while on the other hand you won't be giving your body the fuel it needs to rid itself of these toxins and prevent disease or perform proper healing. It's a no win situation, that can only lead to problems.

We've made the comparison of the human body to an advanced and sophisticated electronic machine. Think of it as something far more advanced, in fact than anything ever created by man. The main factor that sets our bodies apart from anything man-made is its ability to rejuvenate.   This living ability is programmed into every single cell.

An example of this rejuvenating process is seen in what takes place when a bone is broken. This scenario will also show us who and what is really doing the healing.

A doctor cannot make bones mend, no matter how much magical words he pronounces over your break or how many follow-up visits he recommends. Pain killers don't help either.

He may, perhaps be able to set it and to put a splint or cast on, but once that is done, the body takes over. All the "follow-up visits" are merely to put more money in the physician's pocket. The therapy, and medicine that is usually prescribed are only a matter of scheduling what you should be doing for yourself (exercise) or blocking out unwanted symptoms (pain). The true miracle is what is taking place within you.

If you listen to your body, when the pain of a broken bone strikes, then what is the logical thing that you will do? You will rest, of course. Which is exactly what your body needs, a chance to do the work of bringing the broken bones together. Swelling is another symptom that helps the body to perform natural healing functions. When an area of your body swells, it is difficult to move, therefore, that area will get the rest that it probably needs. Fever is another natural mechanism. The first thing most people do when they have a fever is to take aspirin or other fever reducers. But, the body, sometimes only releases needed antitoxins when the temperature is raised. If you turn the heat off, then the body can't do what it must do to heal itself.

This amazing ability of the body to heal itself is seen in even the smallest wounds. If you cut your finger, for instance, the whole body begins to work toward healing the wound. First, pain will signal that there is a problem. Blood will then start to rush toward the cut, to coagulate in order to stop the bleeding. Gradually, a fine scab will form and beneath this the healing process continues. Later, when the scab falls off (usually at exactly the right time) and new tissue has formed where the cut used to be. There was no need for medication or even a bandage. This simplified description of the healing process of a tiny cut does not take into account the myriad systems that are put into effect to combat infection and to close the wound. This is the absolutely amazing ability of our bodies to follow the Creator's plan of action.

The human body, unlike the man-made machine, is gifted with this instinctive power to heal itself, restoring its organs to perfect health, if it is fed the proper fuel. A car that is made to operate on Premium unleaded gasoline, can only function at its peak capacity if it is given the proper fuel. We should not treat our bodies with any less respect than we treat our cars.

It is reported by natural healing doctors that the moment you stop eating unnatural foods and begin nourishing yourself with natural human foods or High Quality Nutrition, your body will begin to alter the course of your health INSTANTLY, and gradually reverse any problems that you might have. Just think how much better than a car or the most sophisticated and advanced computers this is! Our old auto will not be able to run well after having water dumped into the fuel. And, how well will your computer operate if you turn off its source of power?

But, our bodies are very forgiving. Humans can pollute themselves with alcohol and tobacco for years, then if they are smart enough to quit and change their habits they can live as though they never took a drink or a smoke, with almost no ill effects.

The body, by receiving the correct fuel, will employ everything in its power to mend deteriorated and damaged organs and revitalize and rejuvenate the whole body. If you continue to eat only the right foods and give your body the proper nutrition, then your newly revitalize organs can begin working together to harmoniously restore supreme health to the entire system. The evidence of this you can see for yourself with indisputable energy and an extreme vitality. Give your body a chance to show you what it can do. Before you know what is happening, your body will begin to reverse the effects of all negative forces, including aging.

In simple words, after feeding your body with natural foods or High Quality Nutrition for a reasonable amount of time, you will start to grow younger.

Many people who are completely on natural human foods or High Quality Nutrition have reported that they've gained back their youth. Even people in their fifties, sixties and seventies who lived most of their lives eating conventional foods have claimed that they've gained back their faculties, including physical, sexual and mental, to a comparable level they possessed when they were much younger. This is because all of the old and worn out cells of every organ in their bodies have been given new life. Remember, an old HEALTHY person is far better off than a young UN-healthy one.

This is the ONLY doctor that your body usually ever needs. By simply improving the fuel that you supply your body, you can examine this amazing claim for yourself. This is your body and your life we're talking about. Wouldn't you do as much for your car, or any other machine that you might deem important?

Again, we want to emphasize that the same protections that were built into the human body have been built into all life, by the Creator. Just as we have the ability to take care of our individual health, the Earth itself can repair much of the damage that we've done to it...IF we give it the help it needs. We are responsible for the health of the whole earth, just as the Doctor Within Us is responsible for our individual health. In both cases, large and small, the plan is simple, beautiful and workable. We have no right to oppose it.

CHAPTER TWELVE

MOTHER EARTH

Since the beginning of time, we have had the image of our Earth as our Mother and the Spirit of God as Our Father. It did not take a genius to see that there was a natural order of things in the Universe, just as there was a natural order within the framework of our own lives.

Even before we became 'civilized' (and took on the role as the most destructive creatures that ever existed), we had enough sense to see that human life was organized around certain principles. There was an order and balance in the way that things were born or came into being. We observed that seeds grew into trees and eggs produced a variety of life, each species had its own way to produce its own kind. And, we were not different.

In other words, we saw that to **have human life,** we needed a father and a mother. Each parent supplied an essential element in the overall existence of the child. Without the joining of the father and the mother, there was no **procreation.** And we also saw, that the responsibility for the newborn didn't end with birth. Even after a child was born, it was dependent on its parents for survival and learning, to ages beyond those required by other species.

There is, as a matter of fact, a fascinating DUAL character about our humanness. There is something very **special** as well as something FRAGILE about human life. It takes a lot to MAKE a person, but without ALL the essential parts, we don't have anything very special in the least. Without a knowledge of our 'spirit', for instance, we would be just like the other animals. Without a conscience and a caring about others, we would not be fit to act as 'caretakers' for the whole earth.

This image of 'mankind emerging from the earth' is one that we cannot over stress. In Scripture we have noted that 'man was made from the dust of the ground.'We say that the image can be taken even farther than this. We would point to the Native Americans, who call the Earth their Mother and tell you that no more appropriate description for our relationship with the earth can be found. We were literally 'given birth' by the earth itself.

It is obvious that the earth is a living entity. Viewed from space, there is something special about the planets, but especially the earth. While the others look as though they are dead or in the process of being born, the earth sparkles with a brilliance and color that is unknown in any other place in our galaxy. If this tiny planet were not precisely situated where it is in the solar system, then life as we know it could not exist. It is neither too hot, nor too cold. Our winters on the average have not been too long nor our summers too dry. There is also variety on Earth and, like any living creature our planet goes through changes that resemble 'moods' as the year progresses.

The Earth then is without a doubt alive. And, she is responsible for our very existence. We are nourished by the earth daily. Without our Mother's unyielding love for us and continuous care and nurturing, we could not survive even a single day.

Just as a newborn must suckle at its mother's breast, and rely on her for warmth and other protection, we are totally dependent on the Earth for our life's food and sustenance.

It's a wonder and a beauty to behold as we look at the grace and gentleness with which the Earth cares for us. It is also a marvel to see that the same laws that turn the planets in their orbits and the solar systems in their galaxies also govern our own lives and the lives of the most insignificant creature on earth with the same guidance. This order only serves to prove that the laws of nature are far beyond the control of mankind. They are predestined by a much Higher Power.

So it is with the image of the family. This simple unit (father+mother=rebirth) is a pattern that we dare not oppose.

Within this structure is a basic appreciation and respect that is due to our parents. We have continuously told you of our respect for the Creator (or father). We felt an obligation to stress our respect and RESPONSIBILITY to the Earth (our mother) in this chapter.

We cannot, we believe do any justice to the subject of an individual's health without demonstrating how **much** we depend on our Mother Earth for the results we can expect in any health objectives.

Let's look more closely at how the laws of nature have ordained that the relationship of a mother to her child is EXACTLY THE SAME as our relationship with the Earth.

As our knowledge of the processes involved in giving birth increases, we begin to understand a definite cause and effect relationship between the health of the mother and that of her children.

Modern day moms are told not to smoke cigarettes, drink alcohol or take drugs because the odds of their having an effected offspring is greatly increased.

Women who are alcoholics and drink heavily while pregnant will give birth to alcoholic children or ones who have already been damaged by that drug in some way.

The same is true of mothers who are addicted to drugs. A recent documentary entitled, "<u>What Mother Takes...Baby gets</u>," proves beyond a shadow of a doubt that addicted moms have babies who are just as addicted to drugs as they are.

In graphic video pictures we see newborn babies going through withdrawal from drugs. These babies **ALSO** have many of the other diseases and degenerations associated with drug abuse. Many of them are born with hearing and sight problems. Some have serious brain damage or other life-long diseases. Those who are severely effected usually grow up more slowly and develop less than the children of mothers who did NOT use drugs when they were pregnant.

More and more evidence is being uncovered that shows just how important it is for a mother to remain clean and healthy during her pregnancy.

We are also learning that many of our newest diseases (the results of unnatural lifestyles or contact with a polluted environment) such as AIDS or cancer or diseases of the liver, kidneys or other organs, can all be passed directly from the mother to the child BEFORE IT TAKES ITS OWN FIRST BREATH!

This is a sad but increasingly common story for people in the modern world. On a much more grand scale, we can say that ALL OF US have been born of a mother who is growing more ill by the day. The irony is that WE have made our mother sick.

And, the harder she tries to nurture us, the more she gives us of herself, the more difficult it is for her to survive on her own.

Look how this translates into what we have done to our own earth. WE have caused the sickness of our mother by polluting her with chemicals, by cutting her forests and by disrupting her at every chance we have in her efforts to make herself well. We have gone so far as to strip the protecting layers of clothing (the Ozone Layer) and other protections that exist so that our Mother has no immunity from the shameless destruction that we inflict upon her.

This is just plain stupid, since, by the laws of nature, when our mother is sick then WE will be sick as well. And, not only are we BORN sick (already affected by the pollutions and diseases that we ourselves have created) but we continue to abuse our mother and make it impossible for her to nurture us and care for us the way she is driven to.

How have we allowed our 'family' to be broken and destroyed in such a manner? Why have we stood by and watched as our own mother (our life's blood) was being stripped, raped and murdered? Our only excuse has been that 'we didn't know.'

That, in itself is a shameful lie. Since MANY **DID** know what was happening and simply did nothing or said nothing (or worse yet) lied to the others who were truly ignorant. In this category, the 'wise scientist' is again brought to mind. This character, in the evil guise of someone trying to 'improve upon creation', has helped to camouflage the truth about our mother's condition for the welfare of his own bank account.

We were kidnapped from our mother's bosom and told by our captors that THEY were responsible for our well-being and health. We were told to ignore the voice of our father and to remove ourselves from an association with our mother. We were kept from any contact with our parents by the scientists as they filled our free time with worthless pursuits and our heads with needless facts.

When we heard the call of the Inner Voice to return to nature (our mother) our Impostor Parents (Science and Technology) said, "Ignore that voice. You don't want to take a walk in the forest. Here, watch this television. It will give you all the knowledge you need."

When we were hungry and wanted an apple the Impostor Parents said, "Don't eat a plain apple. It isn't big enough or red enough. Here, let me spray it with chemicals and pump some more chemicals into the ground near the tree. "

We were promised miracles and were given emptiness and disease, both for ourselves and our mother earth.

But, this is the story on the surface. What lies beneath is even more evil and insidious. For, the truth is that all these doings were based upon a single sin, the **Sin Of Greed for MONEY!**

In an attempt to find more ways to fool the general public, Science and Technology went straight to the source that nurtures us all. They went straight at the jugular of the Mother Earth. About fifty years ago our full efforts to reap a profit were thrust DIRECTLY into the earth itself. Coal, oil, Uranium and other natural resources became our main concern.

Like a good mother, the earth (at first) gladly gave what she had. But, then our greed became too great, our methods too threatening. To get a jewel off our mother's finger, we started cutting off her hands. To drink her milk, we drained her blood.

Then, to fill the void we created with the many holes we'd dug, we started pouring chemicals and other wastes into the soil and waterways. Our production of chemical wastes was so extreme that, in a short time, we had refilled all the holes we had made and were looking for NEW holes to fill with our plastic/chemical toxics. We saw a valley, we filled it up. We discovered a canyon....we filled it to the brim with plastic bleach bottles and hefty trash bags.

Even the ocean was not large enough to contain our species' discards. Pollution now can be found at every depth in all the seven seas.

Were the Impostor Parents angry with themselves for creating such a mess? No! Even today they continue to praise their work and scorn nature, pointing our attentions **away** from our in-bred desire to help our Mother Earth and toward meaningless statistics that show that their profit margin has steadily increased 3% and that unemployment is down.

If a robber was beating your mother in your living room, would you take the time to wonder what was on television ? Of course not! But, that is essentially what has been taking place for the past one hundred years. And, it's not that we are BAD, it's just that we are lazy and have allowed ourselves to ignore what our eyes are telling us. Certainly we see that our mother is being beaten. But, we have been told not to believe what we see for so long (and only listen to what our Impostor Parents are telling us) that we assume that our own Inner Voice is wrong and that what we're being told is the Truth.

The true horror lies in the fact that we not only have allowed ourselves to be fooled, but we have sat by while 'THE PROCESS OF LIFE' and the order of the Universe has been killed as well.

Now our Mother is Sick and is fighting for her own life, and we are being born sick as she continues to try and give us life.

The examples of this perversion are in the tiniest microorganisms that exist in our soil, air and water. These creatures, invisible to our naked eyes, are as alive as the earth itself. They are also children of the Mother Of Us ALL, and are fed and nurtured by her.

In return, these tiny organisms help to keep the soil alive by returning their own bodies and their NATURAL waste to it. These microorganisms are an important enriching element for any other life forms that thrive on the earth. They play an important role in nourishing the vegetation that is grown in a particular soil. When we put chemical fertilizers (poisons) into our soil, we usually kill these tiny life forms. We used to tell our own children, "don't eat meat; don't eat dairy products; eat more vegetables and fruits." But in our own life time the situations have all changed. When the soils that we use to grow our produce is toxic due to pesticides and acid rain, then what shall we tell our children to eat? In the end, we ALL suffer.

We need to stop and examine our priorities. Is the car and television set so important to us that we will sacrifice our own health, the health of our planet AND the health of all our children?

Our scientists would love to go to places like Hunza and Vilcabamba and teach these people how to modernize and improve their lives. But, if we examine how closely this modernization will translate into an inferior food, then it would serve these same scientists if they went to these places NOT to teach, but to LEARN.

A recent SPECIAL EDITION of 20/20 on ABC television, posed the question, Imagine being 130 years old and playing tennis. Well why not?" The show was called "Slowing Down The Clock." It was about the NEW possibility of living to 130 years of age IN PERFECT HEALTH (something that we've been saying all along). This particular segment made many suggestions that were, in our opinion very truthful and honest. What they DIDN'T do, was go ALL THE WAY. The information that was made available from this program led the viewer to believe that MORE fiber and vegetables was good and LESS meat, dairy products and fat etc. would also benefit an individual. While these kinds of statements are certainly true, they are not THE WHOLE TRUTH. Remember, we can't have a healthy cell without a healthy body; just as we can't expect to have healthy individual species without taking care of the whole environment.

In our overly industrialized society, we put chemical fertilizers in the soil, we add more chemicals to our foods after we spray them with pesticides and then we feed these same chemical-rich grains and greens to our livestock. And, if that is not enough WE EAT this livestock AFTER we accelerate their growth and 'improve' their fitness for our purposes, by shooting them full of more chemicals in the form of steroids, hormones and antibiotics. All these chemicals are transferred to our own systems once we partake of the animal's flesh or its products (eggs and milk for instance).

We might think that we are doing the earth a favor by meddling with the laws of nature, but we really aren't. In the end, our intrusions have made it difficult for us to do anything about rescuing ourselves.

What is particularly interesting is that, EVEN NOW our Mother Earth has not abandoned her love for us. With all that we've done and continue to do to ensure her total destruction, our Mother continues to try and care for us, in the best possible way.

What can we do? Again, we must stop and look to the Super Healthy Communities of the world. These people have NOT so disrupted the natural laws that their foods are nutritionally worthless. Their soils are cultivated, their foods harvested according to the highest standards of the natural processes. Their soils are also completely free of chemicals and are highly fertile and filled with microorganisms and minerals (necessary for a rich harvest). In addition, their clean air, water, sun and other natural elements help produce food with FULL NUTRITIONAL VALUE. These are the places where humans live in harmony with their Earth Mother and treat her with the respect she deserves. This ensures a high level of HEALING potency from every bite. Their food, therefore is not only nourishing, but gifted with HEALING POWER.

Our world has become one of **import and export**. When we have a need, there is always someone who can fill our orders. We spend the money to import televisions and cars from Japan and clothing from Taiwan. We get our leather goods from Italy and Spain and other goods from any other part of the world that can and will provide them. Why don't we get our FOOD from such a place?

Rather than end this chapter with a question, we thought it would be fitting to give you a few statistics earth's health as we did about your own health in an earlier chapter.

To close this book on a positive note we've offered a few suggestions for things YOU can do to aid the Earth in it's struggle to cleanse itself.

NUMBER OF RAIN FOREST ACRES BEING DESTROYED

50 PER MINUTE

COUNTRY WHICH PRODUCES THE MOST POLLUTION WHICH CAUSES GREENHOUSE EFFECT

United States (causes one fifth of all global pollution)

AMOUNT OF MONEY SPENT BY ALL NATIONS ON DEFENSE

One Trillion dollars annually

AMOUNT NEEDED FOR ENVIRONMENT

ADDITIONAL $150 BILLION A YEAR

WHAT YOU CAN DO TO HELP THE EARTH

1) Insulate your home and weather strip the windows. If possible, use high efficiency glass and set air conditioners at a reasonable temperature.

2) Avoid toxic household and garden chemicals. Vinegar and lemon juice works as well as many cleaners and they don't pollute.

3) Use the LOWEST WATTAGE possible for every light bulb. You might not need a 150 watt in every case. If a 40 watt will do, then use one.

4) Make BIODEGRADABLE a test word for all your purchases. LOOK AT LABELS. To determine whether a substance is toxic or non-biodegradable look at the label.
5) Biodegradable also means using cloth diapers instead of plastic ones OR a new alternative is a biodegradable disposable kind that can be purchased at most health food stores.

6) RECYCLE everything possible.

7) Don't drive alone when you can ride with someone else and don't drive at all when you can walk or ride a bike.

8) Don't WASTE anything (especially water).

9) VOTE FOR THOSE WHO HAVE PROVEN THEY CARE ABOUT HEALTH AND THE ENVIRONMENT.

CHAPTER THIRTEEN

OTHER IMPORTANT POINTS TO CONSIDER

The Value Of Organic Food

We have already mentioned some of the benefits regarding Organically Grown food from a physiological standpoint.   It is important to remember that foods grown naturally through organic methods are far superior to commercially grown food. This matter is so important that we want to emphasize this to you once again. We recommend that you learn to grow your own organic vegetables if possible, or purchase them when available and affordable. Here we want to talk about organic foods from the standpoint of their therapeutic value. There is much more to buying organic foods than just the nutritional value (which is far superior to commercially grown produce). That value comes in the ability that the organic food has in 'putting us in touch with our own roots.'

By this we mean, to grow a tree and see it bear fruit; THEN to feel the life giving force that the fruit yields when we use it for food. THIS is keeping in touch with the life force itself. And,this is another big bonus to eating organically grown fruits and vegetables.

In addition, there is a certain amount of work (that's physical labor) involved in growing foods organically. As you now are aware (from your reading of the Ten Health Commandments), exercise is a necessity for Ultimate Health. This is one exceptionally fine way to get your exercise AND be a part of the natural process. Growing your own vegetables and fruits is a pastime that many consider equal to any meditation.

Starting Method (Revolutionary or Gradual)

When you finally decide that you've had enough of your old life's aches, pains and disease, (we hope that we've convinced you that the best time is NOW) you are going to have to make that very important first decision.. That choice is ALL important because it could, at the outset, determine whether you will succeed or fail.

What you need to decide is HOW you are going to start your program toward your ultimate health. According to the research that we've done, there are essentially only two choices. Here they are. Look them over. Think about which is best for you and then, choose well based upon what you (and your inner voice) know about the kind of person that you are.

Revolutionary: You can think of your decision to change your lifestyle toward good health as a personal revolution. This revolution for good health can begin by you deciding to eliminate 'over night' all unnatural foods from your diet. Then, from that moment on, you must eat only according to the recommendations of this book and adhere to the "Ten Commandments of Hunza Superior Heath". The advantages of this method are many, not the least of which is that the sooner you change the balance of health in your diet from Toxic and Unnatural to Natural and Healing, then the better off you will be in every area. Many people have achieved wonderful results by exercising a little will power. You can too.

We offer this caution however. If you choose the revolutionary method as the course you will take, you must prepare yourself for a sudden change in the body's cleansing mechanism. NOT ALWAYS, but with some people, this will result in a variety of very brief and temporary discomforts. These brief periods of discomforts vary in severity and length of time, and are usually a good sign, meaning that your body is flushing out the toxic wastes. Individuals with very serious health problems may even experience a temporary set back in their recovery. Then, the improvement will be incredibly fast. Don't worry or revert back to your old habits unless the reactions are EXTREME or last for long periods of time without any signs of improvement in any area.

Gradual: If the above scenario frightens you to the point that you don't want to even TRY getting healthier, you may want to choose a slower method to change your diet. This method might also be appropriate for those who try the Revolutionary method but fail at it.

This course is based upon the assumption that the goal of the revolutionary method is the ONE and only real goal for the health seeker. It just tricks your subconscious into thinking that change isn't happening, since it takes place over a longer period of time. For this method you will have to plan and organize a schedule of eliminating the unnatural and toxic food items in your diet over a limited period of time, suited to your needs. The advantage of this method is that it accepts the fact that all people are INDIVIDUALS and must march to the beats of many different drummers. And, as we've stated before, any progress (even slow) is better than none.

The disadvantage of this method is that some people become content with first signs of health results. A little improvement, in some cases is often much better than expected. Therefore, these people do not continue the course to the ultimate goal of a complete natural food diet. Not doing so is hazardous, since it does not remove the possibility of any major or degenerative disease. We look at this stage as climbing HALF WAY UP A MOUNTAIN, when you are perfectly able to make the entire climb. This same problem is also implied, by the way, for those who decide to follow only a FEW of the Health Commandments. What generally happens is that we end up with Commandment Gurus. These are people who find such a change from their old life by following only one or two Commandments, that they forget there are others. An example of this kind of person is the Exercise Nut. This person is one who has found that they can retain a high level of health for extended periods simply by exercising. The truth is that exercise, added to a life that has never experienced it before WILL help to improve it radically. BUT, the change for the better is NOT ultimate health. ALL the Health Commandments must be adhered to for this to occur.

You must, therefore, be willing to take the responsibility for the dangers of the Gradual method and stick to your chosen plan up to the end of the schedule. A sample elimination schedule is given at the end of this chapter for your reference. Please use it as a guide on your journey to health.

The Ins and Outs of Fruit

Again, we have already outlined a number of positive attributes to fruits in a Hunza Health Life-style. A couple of additional comments we wanted to add are:
1) Most people do not know that the outer layers of fruits and grains have a high degree of nutritional content. The skins of some fruits and most grains provide "roughage" which helps solve many health problems including those associated with the digestive system and heart.
2) There has been some recent scares in the media dealing with the high level of toxicity in the skins of fruits (especially apples). You must be careful, but NOT paranoid.
3) Even if you THINK that your fruit is organically grown, it is important to thoroughly wash it to remove very dangerous chemicals which may have been sprayed on the fruit by commercial growers. An additional caution is in order. Since these chemicals can be absorbed into the fruit, it is best to eat organically grown fruit if available and affordable. Of course, if you've grown your own vegetables and fruits from seeds,then you'll KNOW that they are O.K. In this case, EAT THE SKIN. It tastes good and it's GREAT for you.

Half-Empty

Human beings are animals of instinct and reflex to a large degree. And, like all other animals, we function better (our senses are keenest and reactions sharpest) when it is NECESSARY. It is only logical that our bodies would respond best to food, when they are not completely full.

Our advice then is, no matter how many times a day you may eat, try not to overdo it. This is a much more natural way of eating. Overeating is a habit which people in a modern life have conditioned themselves to. And once conditioned to overeating, it is most difficult to overcome.

One of the most sage pieces of advice on the subject comes from the oriental teachings which suggest, "Eat enough to fill your stomach 1/3 full. Drink enough water to fill another 1/3 and leave the final 1/3 empty." We would add that it would probably do you no harm, if you left up to 1/2 of your stomach empty at all times.

Chew, Chew, Chew

Here is another example of how Grandma and Grandpa were giving good advice that we thought was silly. We now know that our life-style promotes a far too fast pace in our eating habits. We should all take some time and learn to chew slowly and completely small amounts of food. This will help you properly digest your meal. You will also find that it is a natural way to control your appetite. In addition, you will find that many foods seem to taste 'better'. This will be due to two factors. One is that, as your taste buds become detoxified, they will 'come to life' as the rest of your body will. Also, when you take more time to chew, naturally the experience of actually 'tasting' your food will be totally new for some.

Studies have shown that a final benefit can be reaped by those who change to natural foods or High Quality Nutrition because people who take time in their activities (such as eating) tend to live longer due to less stress. When you make the habit of eating a pleasant ritual then it will lose its stressful connotations in your life. This will be one less thing you 'worry' about and one more thing to enjoy to the fullest.

Stomach Time

There is no special time schedule for eating in a natural lifestyle. In our primitive ancestry, eating took place throughout the day except when we were asleep. The Hunza Health Commandments suggest to "eat when hungry and sleep when tired." Just remember to eat what you feel like and when you feel like it. But limit your choice to only what is recommended in this book.

Another way of attacking this problem would be to seek guidance from yourself. Don't eat because your old habits are motivating you. Be honest with yourself and eat only when 'the spirit' moves you.

Backward motion

We are assuming that those of you who are reading this book have not had the best health habits before now. So, most of the habits that you have are deeply ingrained in your psyche. Do not be discouraged then, if, once in a while, you slip into old habits. Remember we have all become addicted to eating unnatural foods. It took you a long time to develop your habits. It will be hard to give them up. But, as you continue to feed your body with natural foods and High Quality Nutrition the cravings for old unhealthy food will begin to lessen then (one day) vanish completely. Be encouraged by your daily progress. Even a small step forward brings you closer to total good health.

By the same token, don't be disheartened if you do not see progress everyday, or if you seem to stay at the same level for a while. Try to think about how you ONCE WERE, and how YOU WILL BE, not about your lack of apparent movement.

Evaluation of the Hunza Diet

There will be a point in time when you will want and NEED to see some results. If you use a revolutionary approach you can evaluate the full results of this diet in six to nine months from the starting date. This is a relatively short time when we consider the many decades that we have pushed purely toxic materials into our systems. For the more gradual method you must wait six to nine months AFTER reaching the end of your elimination schedule. This will allow enough time for a fair evaluation, although some people see results much sooner. We must stress that individual levels of toxicity, age and genetic factors all play important roles in the rate of your progress. The six to nine month estimates are based on 'averages' of the personal experiences of those who've tried this diet, thus far.

Finally, if you see dramatic results in two or three weeks don't be surprised. We have seen testimonials of some who have experienced amazing results in the first week, but this is not usual.

Healthy Reactions

One final consideration. We've made many comparisons in this book and one that we've used repeatedly is between our bodies and machines. This comparison is valid, but only to a point. Your body is a

LIVING machine. When you begin to eat Natural Human Foods or High Quality Nutrition, you will be putting the cleansing mechanism into full swing to expel the toxic wastes built up over the years from eating unnatural food. Some will be removed quickly. Others may take much longer. The body will react differently for each individual but the likelihood is that the cleansing operation will cause a variety of discomforts.

Do not become alarmed at such healthy reactions as: diarrhea, headaches, stomach aches, fatigue, muscle soreness, sleeplessness or other symptoms. It is very important that you DO NOT take any medication (unnatural substances) for these symptoms. These periods of discomfort will not last long. And, the length of time that you will feel them will only be prolonged if you continue to pollute your system.

Depending on the type of toxic waste deposit and through which system (digestive or respiratory) it is being expelled, the temporary problems will be experienced only with that part of the body affected. Some other minor problems might be bad breath or odor through perspiration on the skin.

Rest and relax whenever it is convenient. Remember these healthy reactions are positive signs, the Hunza Diet is restoring your natural health.

The schedule on the following page is presented as a guide, and a point of reference. You should use it as a resource if you plan to follow the gradual method of eliminating toxic materials from your diet. But, again, don't feel discouraged if you can't follow it exactly. We believe it is a good method of elimination, but there are certainly others. We have prepared the schedule according to the difficulty of dealing with the unnatural foods in question, rather than (in each case) the toxicity level of an individual unnatural food.

This means, for instance, that one of the first things we ask you to do is give up alcohol and coffee. Obviously, white sugar is an even more dead food than coffee, but coffee has the tendency to 'use up' more vitamins than we take in. It, just as alcohol, affects every cell of our bodies 'negatively' rather than being 'merely empty'. Both alcohol and coffee have the added detriment of harming vital organs necessary to the cleansing of the body (such as the liver and kidneys). And, in the case of coffee make all parts of the body work harder and faster to perform at a less healthful level. That is why we have set up our eliminations in the order that we did.

ELIMINATION SCHEDULE
(7 Week Schedule)

Eliminate beginning 1st week:_____
Alcoholic drinks
Coffee

Beg. 2nd week: _____
Soda drinks
Any foods containing chemicals

Beginning 3rd week: _____
Processed food
Desserts

Beginning 4th week: _____

Cake and Ice cream
White flour

Beginning 5th week: _____
Sugar
All fats & animal flesh

Beginning 6th week: _____
Poultry
Fish
Dairy products

Beginning 7th week: _____
Eggs
All Other Offending Foods

(Here we have given you a sample of Elimination Schedule. We suggest you make your own schedule and use as much time as you need.)

CHAPTER FOURTEEN

FINAL WORD

We have come to the point in our book when we must close. This also marks the beginning or your journey toward ultimate personal health. There is a certain amount of anxiety connected with every important decision in life. But, in this case, the goal of total health and well-being make the trip well worth ANY effort.

The tools that you've gained during your reading of the preceding pages, should be enough for you to tip the scales of life in favor of improved health. We believe, that in this book we've offered all the raw materials necessary to combat a conventional life-style. The rest is up to you.

We would like to take this final opportunity to recount what we've discussed, so that there are n o misunderstandings. We also want every reader to be quite clear about where we stand as an organized effort against disease and ill-health practices.

We believe in prevention rather than cure of disease. At the center of this belief is the knowledge that our bodies have been equipped by the Creator with a remarkable ability to repair and take care of themselves. We believe, therefore, that there is truth in this world. And, it is apparent, as well, that we've been granted an infallible method of checking the TRUTH in any situation or question, and that the Creator has given this method a voice that speaks as loudly as we do when we ask the questions. We know the voice of this method as our Inner Voice or our Common Sense, since it is available to us all.

Checking with our Inner Voice, we have come up with some conclusions about the conventional life-style as opposed to one we feel is 'appropriate' for humans. We know, for instance, that our actions as humans have affected every species on earth and are now threatening to destroy the foundations of very earth on which all life is based. This is wrong.

We can see that disease is preventable by looking with an open mind at the great amounts of research on health and vitality that is going on, right now, in our nation, and (more importantly) by examining healthy societies in the world and that the MEANS of prevention are often withheld from us due to greed of individual concerns. This is also wrong.

Along with this, we have seen that the business of "curing" is a huge industry that is generating astronomically high profits for some individuals and organizations. It's ironic that Science and Technology (by their unsavory associations with Business) first work to destroy our very hearts, then when we require a new heart, they put all their efforts into convincing us to buy a new one. Our question is this: Why deteriorate our health to the extent that new organs become necessary? Why not just try to prevent disease? It can be done. This

This book (and the encyclopedia of Common Sense) is filled with proof and evidence.

Our problems arise when we give up our basic human liberties; the liberty to take care of our own bodies and be responsible for our own health. Unfortunately, through years of conditioning, we've given up most of our basic human liberties. The responsibility for our nutrition and health is now in the hands of the farmers. The responsibility of bringing this food to our tables has been turned over to the food manufacturers, processors and market owners. The responsibility of curing disease has been given to physicians, chemical laboratory operators and many other money-making ventures. The power of conditioning and endless advertising results in our ready acceptance of the statements these businesses make about themselves. We accept the absurd claim that doctors can cure disease...as truth, even though (in our hearts) we know that only by following the Creators plan can disease be prevented.

Whatever the moneymongers produce and offer, we eat. Whatever they recommend, we follow. And, sadly, we have allowed most of this to happen in the name of 'convenience' rather than necessity.

By allowing our lives to be dominated by this industrial Profit-making Process we have created the terrifying health corruption that exists today. We have put, not only ourselves but our entire planet in immediate jeopardy. Modern Technology has made the air unfit to breathe, the water unfit to drink, saturated our lives with chemicals and destroyed the very essence of natural sustenance. Advanced Medical Techniques then come to our rescue with more chemicals and other answers at the edge of a surgeon's knife. Neither of these treatments remove the real causes of our diseases. If the true causes are not eliminated then the patient will have recurrences of the same diseases and continued susceptibility to others. And, these are only the physical diseases we are talking about. But the same is true of the emotional and psychological ailments that now run rampant in our modern society.

There is only one proven way to treat the causes of disease. We must take responsibility for following the Natural Laws. We need only to open our minds to the natural processes of life and to use the abundant natural foods available for our well being. We must learn to live within the rules of nature. The primary law is: Give your body the proper fuel for repair and the body will HEAL ITSELF.

The only way we can truly appreciate the preciousness of health is when we are seriously ill. Most of us have experienced some degree of disease which has left us with a need to fight back. Many of us have had to stand by and watch a loved one die of disease. This is one of life's most horrible experiences. What we must realize, however, is that (under the present circumstances) ALL OF US ARE TERMINALLY ILL. Through acceptance of the conventional life-style, we have effectively reduced our lives. We have weakened our health, created stress and anxiety and disassociated our spirits from the Creator's plan.

The GOOD NEWS is that there is STILL HOPE. But, there is very little choice. The only effective way to reverse this negative trend is through natural methods of prevention. The earlier we decide to take action by changing from an unnatural to a more natural eating habit, the sooner we will return to a healthy body. And, since our body is our only true temple, then when we put our HOUSE in order, then the life-style we live and the stresses associated with it will also change for the better. Then, when we feel better, and feel better about ourselves, we can get to the business of healing the earth of the wounds that we've inflicted upon it.

With this in mind, let's ask ourselves a few final questions. First, what is the difference between those of us who believe in Natural Healing (and our supporters) and the ordinary person who is less interested in his health than he is in religiously following the thinking and directions of others?

By way of answering this question, we must raise other queries and examine the possible ways that one might respond. One question is, "Why is there disease?" Another inquiry posses this problem, "Why should a life, which begins (at birth) in perfect health (a gift of creation) later be forced to contend with disease as a normal part of existence?"

As infants, generally, we are brought into existence in perfect health. This is a basic rule of nature. The great exception to this is those children who are born to sick parents.

Whenever we look for an answer 'scientifically' we know that for every effect there is a cause...for every change that takes place, there is a reason. Therefore, for health to change to ill-health, there must be a valid cause or a sensible reason. So much for the scientific perspective.

Let's seek an answer from a religious point of view. Contrary to popular belief, we cannot hold God responsible for our ill-health. The Creator did not intend that the results of his work MUST suffer pain, aches, disease and misery.

The Creator is the profound source of love and compassion, and it is inconceivable that our God, with all His love and compassion would have the WILL to bring so much discomfort, pain, agony and misery to the entire world (and every species) of his creation. To believe this is the same as believing that a father (one with a history of infinite love for his children) would be plotting throughout his life for his children to suffer horrible deaths. This simply doesn't make sense for a loving father and it certainly does not describe our God. We are equally convinced that you do not have such an image of your God either.

Then, why are we told that, "it's the Will Of God" for us to become sick? Because the same people are telling us that, "a doctor can make you well again." No doctor is necessary to help God put things in order. These truths are easily verified by our common sense.

We are too mature (as individuals and as a species) to be fooled into "playing doctor" as we were when we were five or six. The only alternative to pretending that we are unaware of what is going on is to take responsibility for our health.

Obviously, there are some DIRECT responsibilities such as deciding what food to put (or not to put) into our bodies. Then, there are the 'indirect' responsibilities that include polluting the air we breath and allowing circumstances to exist in other parts of the world that I KNOW will affect my air eventually.

Other than these two differences (asking the questions of Why Disease? and How can I take responsibility for my health?) in many ways we, who believe in Natural Healing and our readers share the same feelings and desires as those 'ordinary people' who are less interested in health and indulge themselves in every offending food and habit possible.

We hold ourselves responsible for our health, where another person sees that responsibility as being with his doctor.

As far as we can see, this line of thinking is dangerous, because it gives that kind of person a false sense of righteousness. He thinks that he has the right to go out and do whatever pleases him, because, when the negative results come to light he can simply run to his doctor to correct the mistake.

This relates to a story that occurred last week. A friend had just returned from a heart specialist and said, "I just found out that I have high blood pressure." He went on to explain the strange set of circumstances that ended with this news. "First, I heard that I had kidney stones, " he began. "Then, every six months I had to go to the doctor to break them up and help my body expel them. The last time I was there, the doctor gave me Sodium Bicarbonate, saying that this would prevent the stones from being formed. It is almost a year since I've had problems with kidney stones, but now the Bicarbonate has raised my blood pressure."

I couldn't help asking what took place next. "The original doctor,"continued the unfortunate friend. " Sent me to a heart specialist who is so worried about me that he's prescribed another drug to reduce the blood pressure."

Without any concern for Ultimate Health, we are forced by this story to ask certain new questions. First, which is a worse suffering: Having your Kidney Stones broken up every six months or worrying about high blood pressure and hearth disease? Secondly: What side effect does this drug for high blood pressure have on our friend?

These questions are typically human ones, that must be answered THOUSANDS of times a day, by normal, ordinary people. That is because our friend and all those people just like him have not learned to take responsibility for their health.

A common complaint from people in the same situation as our friend is that it, "doesn't seem like the doctor really understands my problem."

The real problem is that even if the doctor DOES understand the problem and tells our friend what his diet should be and that he should follow the Principles of Health and that if he DOES this he will not need ANY drugs and that the doctor inside him will take care of everything...if all this happened do you think this person would ever go back to that doctor? No, and he probably will continue to run into health problems.

Why? Because this is not what the general public expects from a doctor. And, we usually don't even consider what we don't expect. What we DO expect is that the doctor will take care of us no matter what goes wrong. We are FREE AS A BIRD to do whatever comes to mind to please all of our senses.

The fact is that we are not quite that free. We cannot play with the laws of nature. If we DO play, we must pay for our stupidity...or someone will pay. The laws of creation are God's laws, and we cannot bypass them. If we try the consequences will be severe. And, the payment depends on how serious the 'play' is. (It is appropriate to note that A.I.D.S. is the consequence of serious play with the laws of nature).The payment has gone beyond personal suffering.

On the global level we are now paying for our 'playing' in that we've put all human life in jeopardy. Our payments come and many, varied forms such as narcotics addictions, destruction of the Ozone Layer, pollution of our atmosphere, the threat of nuclear accident and/or War and a host of others, any one of which could result in complete catastrophe for mankind and all life. We have said enough about Gloom and Doom and would prefer to end this book on a brighter note. With a faith in Creation and the Laws of Nature on our side, we can individually regain our health and establish a more natural, pleasant, stress free and happy life for all. In matters of national or global interest, we must join hands in an Organized Effort, dedicated to the perseverance of energies and talents such as ours at the Center to put things back in their proper place.

Our final word is straightforward and simple: **Observe the LAWS OF NATURE, EAT HIGH QUALITY NUTRITION** and follow the **Ten Commandments for "Hunza Superior Health"** and leave the rest to nature. The end result will be **supreme health, vitality and endless energy. This is a very cheap and easy way to gain such valuable treasures.**